Juicing Recipes: 3-Day Detox For Weight loss, Healthier Skin, Energy Boost and Focus

Printed in the United States of America

First Printing, 2015

Big Leaf Publishing
4644 W. Gandy Blvd, #4-181
Tampa, Fl 33611

www.JuiceFam.com

Disclaimer:

This book offers nutritional information and is designed for educational purposes only. You should not rely on this information as a substitute for, nor does it replace, professional medical advice, diagnosis, or treatment. If you have any concerns or questions about your health, you should always consult with a physician or other health-care professional. Do not disregard, avoid or delay obtaining medical or health related advice from your health-care professional because of something you may have read in this book. The use of any information provided on within these pages is solely at your own risk.

If you are in the United States and think you are having a medical or health emergency, call your health care professional, or 911, immediately.

Reviews

This is a great book for those interested in juicing for health, weight loss, and for clearer skin! This book nicely explains why, when, and how to juice. The recipes are easy and delicious! This is definitely worth picking up when you are ready to adopt a juicing lifestyle!
Brandi R. - www.BrandiJRoberts.com

As someone who has tried a few juice fasts before, I can say that this book does a great job of explaining what to do and what to expect. It gave very practical advice for completing a juice fast. Rather than just throwing out a few recipes, like a lot of books do, they went further by giving a schedule along with those recipes so you know when to eat what. I definitely recommend it!
Sandy Donovan - www.ClearlyInfluential.com

I will be ordering this book for a few friends of mine who tend to go overboard on detoxes and can never finish one. The authors provide you with a lot of excellent information and make it easy to follow. They let you know what produce is best to buy organic, give you the shopping lists and recipes. You are even given suggested times to drink the juice. It is a truly doable juice detox and I really appreciate the advice on how to eat before and after the cleanse. I highly recommend this for anyone considering a juice detox cleanse.
Angelica W.

Contents

Free Gift

Hello fellow Juice Fam Team. Before going any further we want to provide you with a complimentary gift to go with this book.

As our way of saying thank you we want to give you **FREE** juicing recipes to help you complete your journey.

To get your **FREE** juicing recipes and become one of our VIP's head over to http://www.juicefam.com/free-updates today!

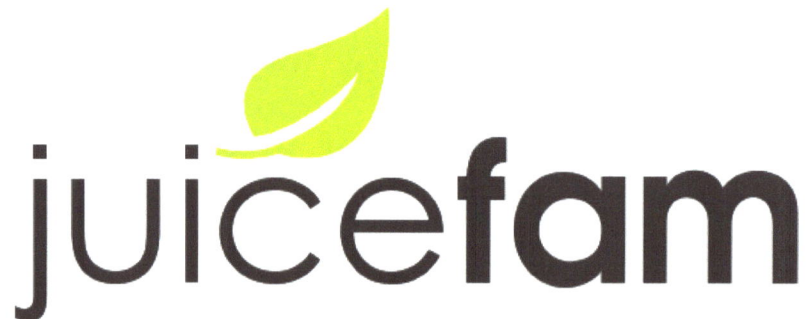

juicefam

Introduction

In the world we live in today, so many people are unhealthy, overweight, and plain out lazy. We won't say it's 100% their fault.

Having access to 24 hour fast food chains on pretty much any street corner and junk food advertised every minute on television makes it very difficult to eat and stay healthy.

Not fueling your body properly can lead to serious health issues and even obesity. Nowadays people eat for pleasure instead of using it as energy as their body intended it for.

Lucky for you, we're also in a time where finding information on natural remedies and good nutrition is only a mouse click away.

We want to share our story with you to show you that with a little guidance and some willpower that you can reverse the same problems we had that you now face.

Let's start off by telling you who we are:

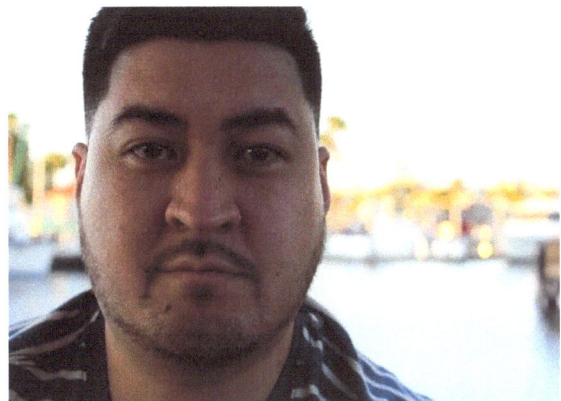

Jimmy is an actor and internet personality from Tampa, Florida. He spent several years working in and running many businesses. Currently working in the

I.T. field and putting so much time and energy into his career didn't leave him much time for eating right or exercising, though, and he knew he had to regain control of his habits and get back into shape.

Jimmy realized that to get ahead and achieve his goals, he would need to make some serious changes.

This is when juicing became an option for him.

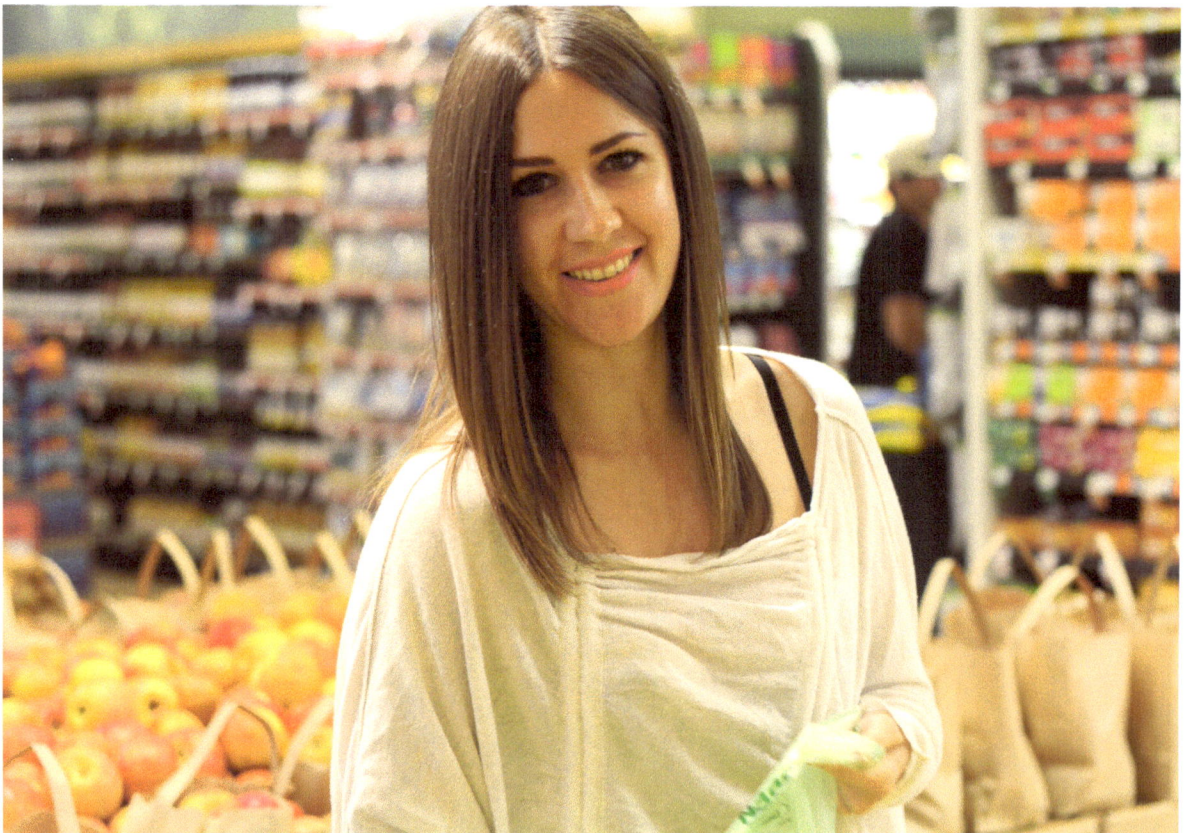

Melissa is a passionate health advocate for all things natural, most importantly the food that we eat.

Now, with Melissa's help, Jimmy has learned how to improve his health through juicing and eating clean. She has shared her knowledge of how to get back to basics with food by removing the toxic preservatives and cooking with fresh whole ingredients.

With her help, he committed to a lifestyle change and now, thanks to everything he learned from her, Jimmy has altered the way he thinks about food and nutrition.

Melissa dedicates her time and passion to health and inspiring others by helping them identify which ingredients to avoid and how those ingredients impact their weight gain, mental state, work-out regimen, and daily routines.

Now together we are both passionate about health and health awareness and have discovered through our own efforts, how to heal from within by choosing organic whole foods, incorporating juicing into our weekly nutrition plans and completing juice/detox cleanses multiple times per year.

We too know what's like to struggle with certain ailments such as - acne, weight gain, bloating, fatigue...etc, and how that impacts our daily lives.

The total embarrassment of experiencing noticeable symptoms and not knowing where to begin to treat them are just some of the things this detox juice cleanse will help alleviate.

Your symptoms, no matter how big or small, are definitely something to pay attention to.
We also understand that these symptoms are our bodies' way of telling us that something is off balance, that something isn't right.

Juicing has changed our lives and we have seen first hand the benefits of what consuming raw fresh vegetable and fruit juice on a consistent basis can do. Through this series of books, we are helping to raise awareness about the importance of your health and the impact that juicing can have on it.

Please use this series of detox cleanses as a stepping stone to jump starting your nutrition plan, or to compliment an already healthy lifestyle, and while your symptoms may not be completely cured within 3 days, feel free to repeat as needed to give your body the recharge it needs.

To make this process as smooth as possible for you, we've done all the hard stuff and taken all the guess work out by compiling an easy 3 day, step by step blueprint written for you on exactly how to detoxify your system via juicing.

The recipes chosen in each volume of our series have specific benefits for your health and while the recipes will all work together as a whole, we've purposely chosen what fruit and vegetable combination will work best for your goals. Whether that goal is to clear up acne, boost your energy, or for weight loss, our tested and proven juice recipes along with detailed instructions will help you achieve the results you are aiming for.

Many other juicing and/or detoxing books out there are just fluffed and hyped with tons of random recipes. If recipes are what you are seeking than that is fine, but if your objective is to detox and goal specific such as losing weight, clearing up your skin, or even boosting your energy, then you've come across the perfect series of books.

By taking that leap and being a part of our 3 day journey you will gain so much knowledge about your body and how it reacts to certain foods, along with learning that you can control how you feel on a day to day basis with just a few minor tweaks here and there in your diet.

We pride ourselves on teaching you from real world experiences and we've outlined a blueprint that will provide you with all the tools and tips necessary to make this process smooth as possible.

Throughout the following chapters, we will walk you through the basics of health and juicing - how to determine which produce is best for your goal, exactly what items to purchase, the equipment you will need, and how to prepare your body for the detox.

Most importantly we will be here 'hand holding' you throughout the detoxification process by coaching you through possible symptoms and assisting with easing back into healthier eating habits once you have completed the cleanse. **So let's get started.**

FAQs

1. FAQ What is detoxing and cleansing?

Basically this is a process by which a person undergoes a program usually involving some diet change or supplement to the diet in order to try to eliminate some of the toxins and parasites that can build up in the body over time.

Factually, we live in a chemical society with numerous potentially harmful chemicals all around us in our environment. They can be in our homes, place of work, shops, restaurants, in fact everywhere. Our bodies are constantly eliminating harmful substances through the urine, bowel movements, sweat and breathing etc.

However, many toxins can remain in the body either lodged in the fat cells or in organs or intestines and it is important to try to help the body from time to time to eliminate these things.

When our bodies become toxic, our natural ways of flushing out metabolic waste from contributing factors such as environmental pollution and an unhealthy diet have exceeded the capacity for what the body can detox on its own. As a result, every system in the human body can become affected. Toxicity makes us sick!

A car can usually run a long time without an oil change but eventually this will cause excessive wear on the engine and the car could start to run poorly. A regular oil change and service can prolong effective operation etc.

Similarly for the body. We recommend a cleanse/detox program should be done at least once, preferably two or even three times each year.

2. FAQ - What are signs that you may need to detox?

These symptoms can come and go, however when they are pretty persistent, it may be a sign that you are building toxicity in the body and need to recharge your system by doing a cleanse.

- Constipation
- Persistent headaches, muscle aches and muscle fatigue
- Food allergies
- Stubborn weight loss
- Skin abnormalities such as acne, rosacea or eczema
- Menstrual problems
- Bloating
- Low-Grade infections

3. FAQ - How long does it take to detox with a juice cleanse?

The process that we will be covering will span a 3 day time frame. Our recommendation is starting this on a Friday and ending it on Sunday evening; this will allow the necessary prep time for your juices and time for monitoring your bodies response system. If you are a beginner to juicing, we believe in the 'less is more' rule by starting with a simple 3 day cleanse. 3 days is an ample amount of time to recharge your system and show improvement with some of the symptoms you may be experiencing. We do not recommend doing a juice detox cleanse for more than 10 days due to the lack of protein and healthy fats that you deprive your body from after long periods of only drinking fruit and vegetable juice.

4. FAQ - Does Juice Cleanses help with weight loss?

Yes absolutely, because you are taking a break from processed meat, heavy starches, wheat, gluten and items that can slow your metabolism down, you will see some weight loss from a cleanse. The state of your nutrition and health before starting a juice detox cleanse will also affect the amount of weight that you will lose. With a 3 day cleanse, typically the majority of the weight lost will be toxins.

5. FAQ - Does juicing remove or reduce acne?

Think of our skin as an alert mechanism. Our skin reacting with acne is our body's way of telling us that something is amiss. There are multiple reasons we can become a victim of acne - hormonal changes, certain medications, stress, toxicity buildup which can block the body's normal regulatory system, and dietary factors, specifically an excess of refined sugars and carbohydrates, dairy products, trans fats and wheat, to name a few. To answer your question, yes juicing can reduce and possibly remove your acne (it completely cleared mine! [Melissa]). Juicing sends a super shot of vitamins, minerals, antioxidants and beta carotene (and the list goes on!) into your body, quenching it with the much needed helpers to get your skin glowing again. Juicing also helps to remove the toxicity buildup in your system which clears everything out.

6. FAQ - Are detox pills the same as juicing?

No. Our personal research has shown us that oftentimes, detox pills contain artificial fructose, dextrose, preservatives and even food coloring in them. All of which can lead to weight gain, diabetes, tumors, allergies...and the list goes on. Your health is ALWAYS better served with a natural detox cleanse. Fruits and vegetables contain the vitamins and minerals needed to support the organs that flush our systems.

Why Organic?

Before we begin this "Why Organic?" section, we want you to know that this book isn't trying to persuade you into going organic or not. We want to educate and inform you that since we are giving you the best possible information and instructions out there on how to perform a three day detox, it is our duty to teach you of the toxins in the fruits and vegetables that are a part of the ingredients in your juicing regimen.

"The body becomes what the foods are, as the spirit becomes what the thoughts are"

Start with the source:

Improving health starts with being informed and educating ourselves with what works for our bodies, what causes certain ailments and disease, and how best to avoid them. It makes the most sense to begin with how we nurture our bodies from within - what is the fuel that we provide ourselves with every day, and what are the long term effects? It goes beyond counting calories and simply observing the food that we eat. To really start with the source, we need to learn about how food is farmed and what is being put into the food that is farmed, how is this food prepared and what is being put into the food that is prepared.

All of these factors add up and greatly affect our health in the long run.

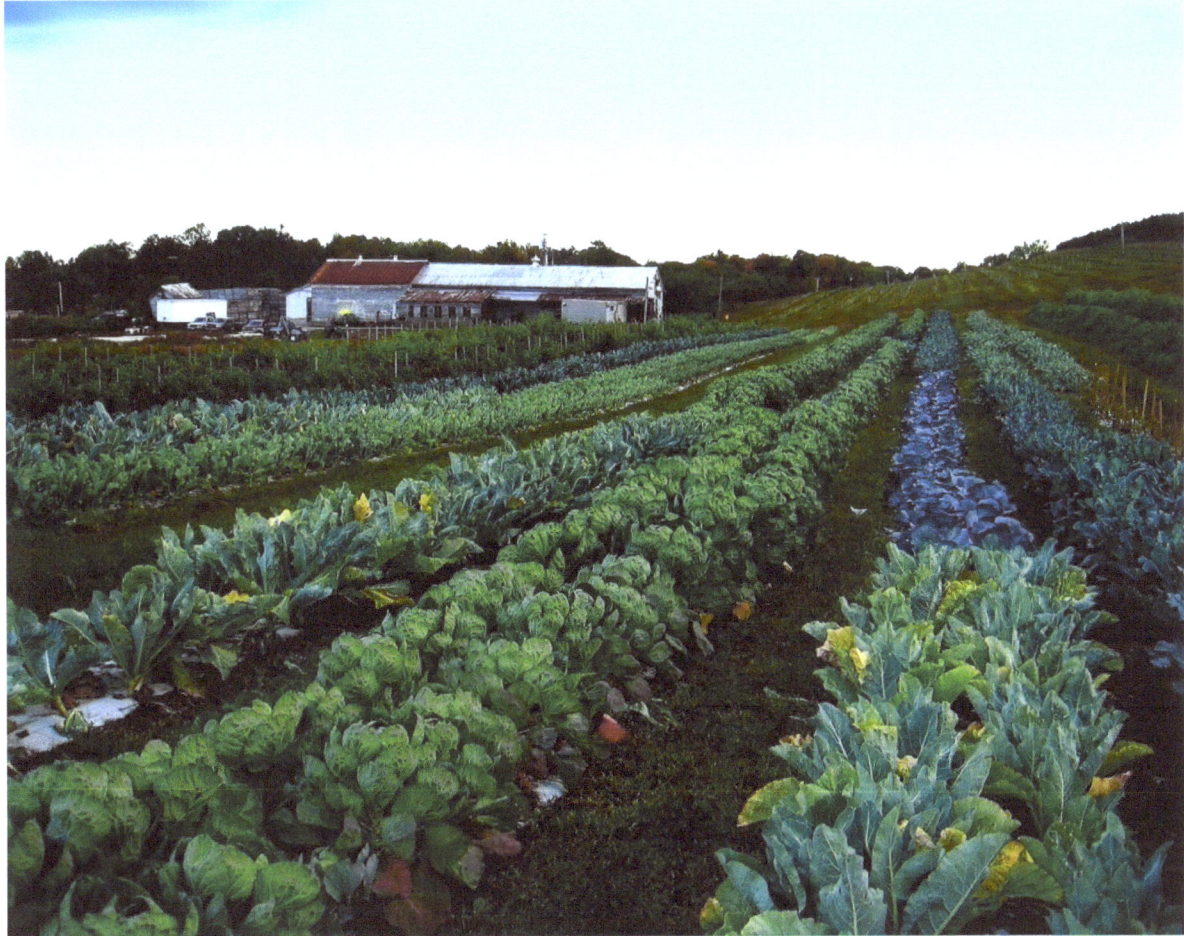

Photo by Amylovesyah

The difference in organic vs non organic farming:

There are major differences in the methods that organic farmers use compared to non organic/conventional farmers. Organic farms rely on a natural eco system that is built which uses crop rotation to alternate the crops grown in each field - this maintains the integrity of the soil naturally. By doing so, they eliminate the need for insecticides in many crops because the cycle of insects are interrupted by the rotation. Certain predatory insects are released onto the farm to control the pests that gravitate toward and destroy the crops that are grown, which eliminates the need for chemical insecticides.

Organic farmers also use animal manure and certain natural fertilizers which help control erosion. Weed management is used versus weed elimination by enhancing crop competition and phytotoxic effects on weeds.

In addition, organic farms strictly limit the use of various methods including synthetic fertilizers and pesticides; plant growth regulators such as hormones, antibiotic use in livestock, GMO's (genetically modified organism) and human sewage sludge.

So how does this affect our health? The answer is simple, if the soil and plants are healthy then WE are healthy.

Non organic farming does not use crop rotation, they grow the same crops in the same location, year after year. Because of this the plants become defenseless, requiring the use of synthetic insecticides to control the pests that destroy the crops. They also require the use of synthetic fertilizers, genetically engineered organisms and growth enhancers to stimulate their soil and crops, resulting in nutrient deficient (inferior) soil.

Know when it's necessary to purchase organic:
When purchasing your fruits and vegetables for your detox, we encourage you to buy organic as this will be the most nutrient dense option. It is not required so if you opt to go non organic, we have included a list of fruits and vegetables that contain the most pesticides, and if you can, please make sure that at least these items are always purchased organic: The Dirty Dozen

Apples	Grapes
Carrots	Kale
Celery	Lettuce
Cherry Tomatoes	Spinach
Collard Greens	Strawberries
Cucumbers	Sweet Bell Peppers

Brief Before, During, and After

Quick Note: we strongly suggest you begin preparing yourself on Monday or Tuesday by slowly cutting back on processed foods and caffeine and then starting your detox on Friday lasting through Sunday.

Now before we dive into your three day journey, there are a few things we need to go over.

How you will feel, what you should be doing throughout these days, and what to do next once it is over.

If this is your first time detoxing, it's important that you understand that your body may be in for a little surprise. Unless you're already living a healthy lifestyle and eating a balanced and clean diet, the withdrawal from not consuming addictive food additives, preservatives, trans fats and sugar can cause a **major disruption** in how you feel.

During your detox it's important that you hydrate with at least 8 glasses of water per day and keep extraneous exercise to a minimum.

While you're finishing your last day and final juice mix for the detox it will be time to get you thinking about whole foods again, and how you will wean yourself into healthier food habits.

Resources

Equipment for Juicing:

Whether you are a beginner or an experienced juicer, it is important to know the difference between the types of juicers so that you make an informed purchase. There are two types of juicers - Centrifugal juicers, and Masticating juicers.

Centrifugal juicers typically separate the flesh of fruits and vegetables from the juice by mashing and spinning them against a metal blade pressed against a mesh filter.

Masticating juicers crush and then mash the fruits and vegetables which usually create the most yield of juice. These juicers are also widely valued because they create the most nutrient dense juice for you as there is less heat involved, which doesn't spoil the nutrient content of your juice. You typically spend more money to purchase a masticating juicer for this reason.

We personally have used centrifugal juicers for years and have had phenomenal results, and would recommend you start with one of these juicers if you have never juiced before so that you minimize your investment while easing into juicing. The personal choice is yours, and we have listed examples of these below for your convenience.

In addition, we have listed other helpful items such as cleaning brushes, storage glasses with airtight lids, a cutting board and knife. Everything you need to get started can also be found on our webpage by clicking here: Juice Fam Shop - (http://www.juicefam.com/shop)

Centrifugal Juicer:

Black & Decker JE2200 400-Watt Fruit and Vegetable Juice Extractor with Custom Juice Cup

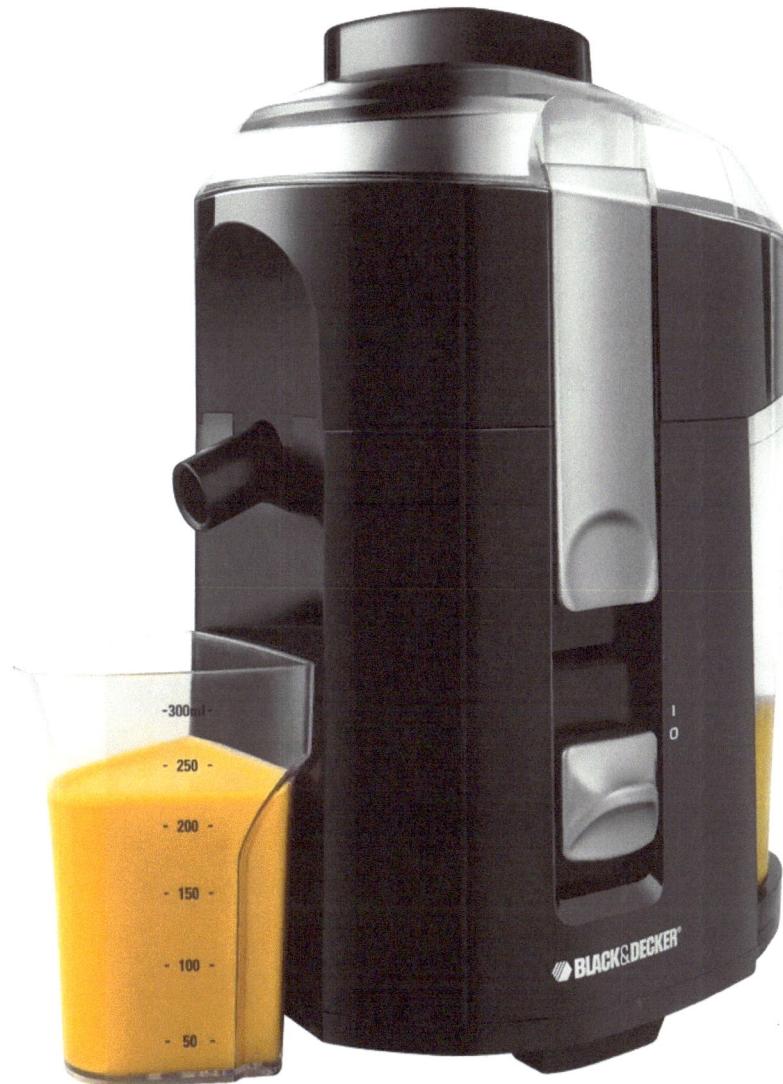

Masticating Juicer:

Breville BJS600XL Fountain Crush Masticating Slow Juicer

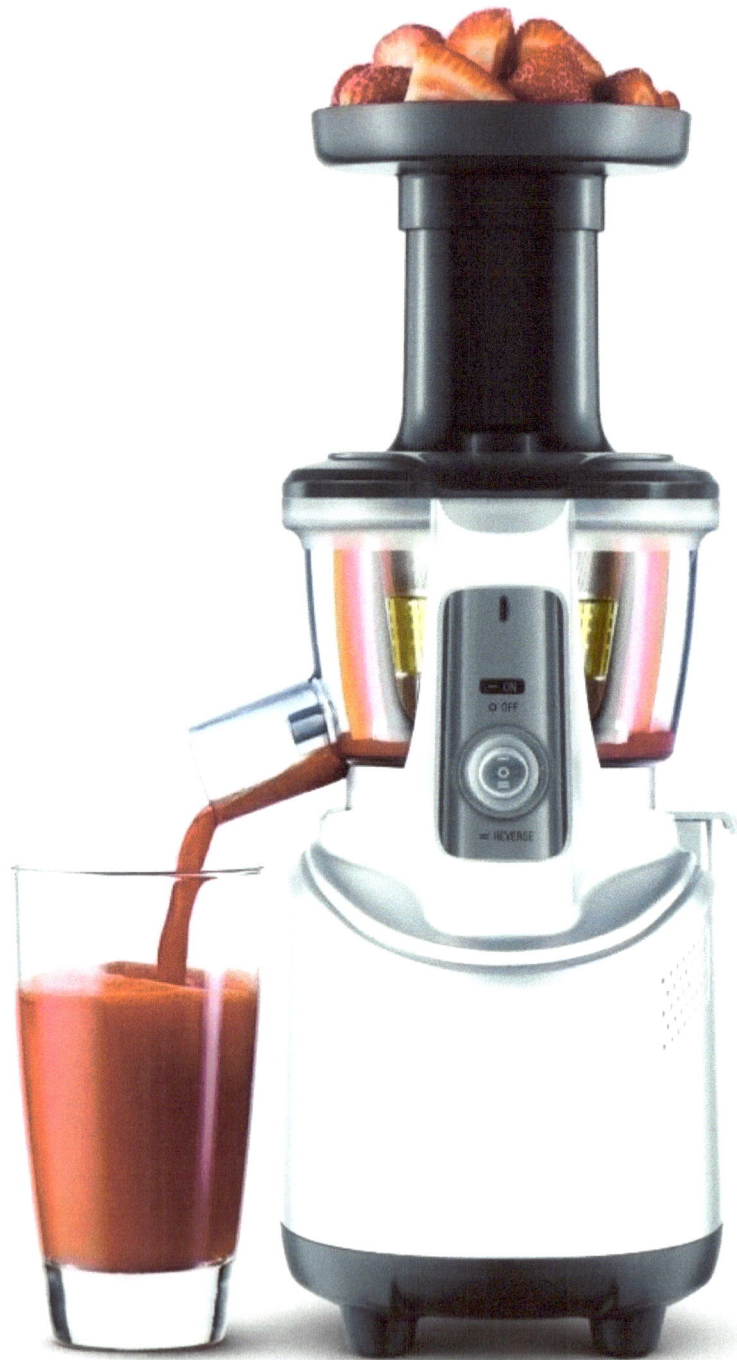

Vegetable Brush:

Bürstenhaus Redecker 5.3-inch Hard and Soft Side Vegetable Brush

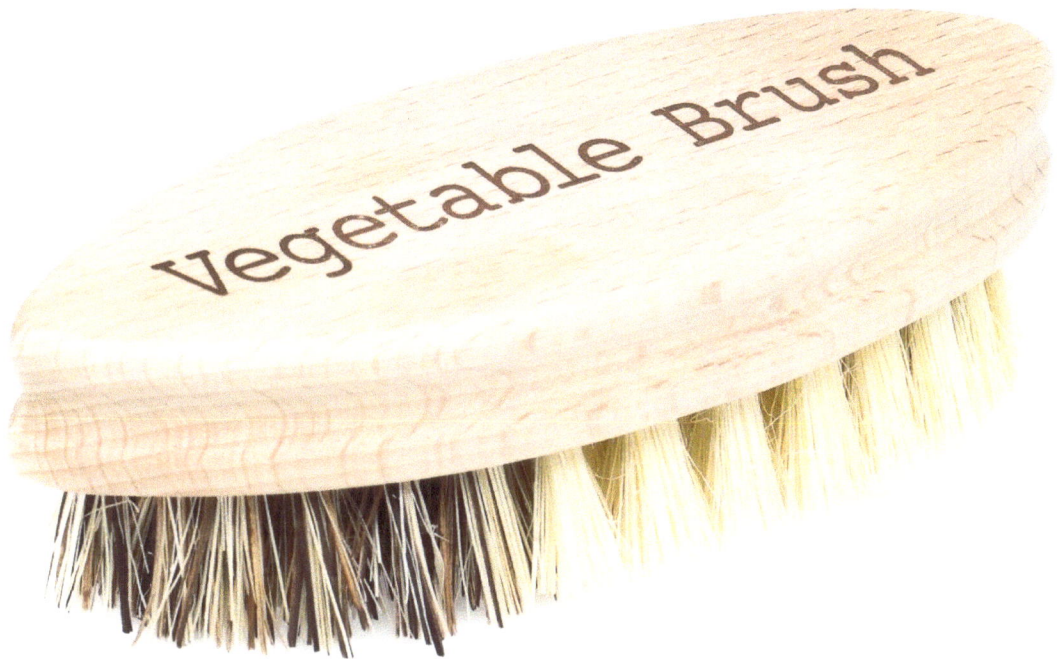

Storage Glass:

Ball wide mouth quart jar

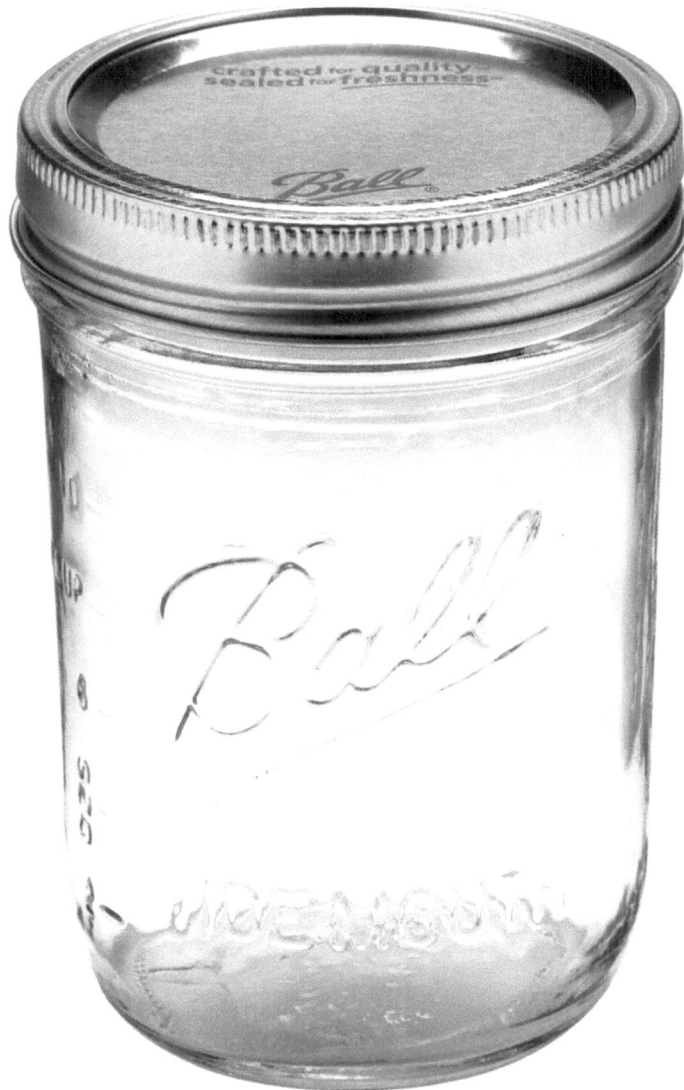

Cutting Board:

Extra Thick Bamboo Cutting Board Set

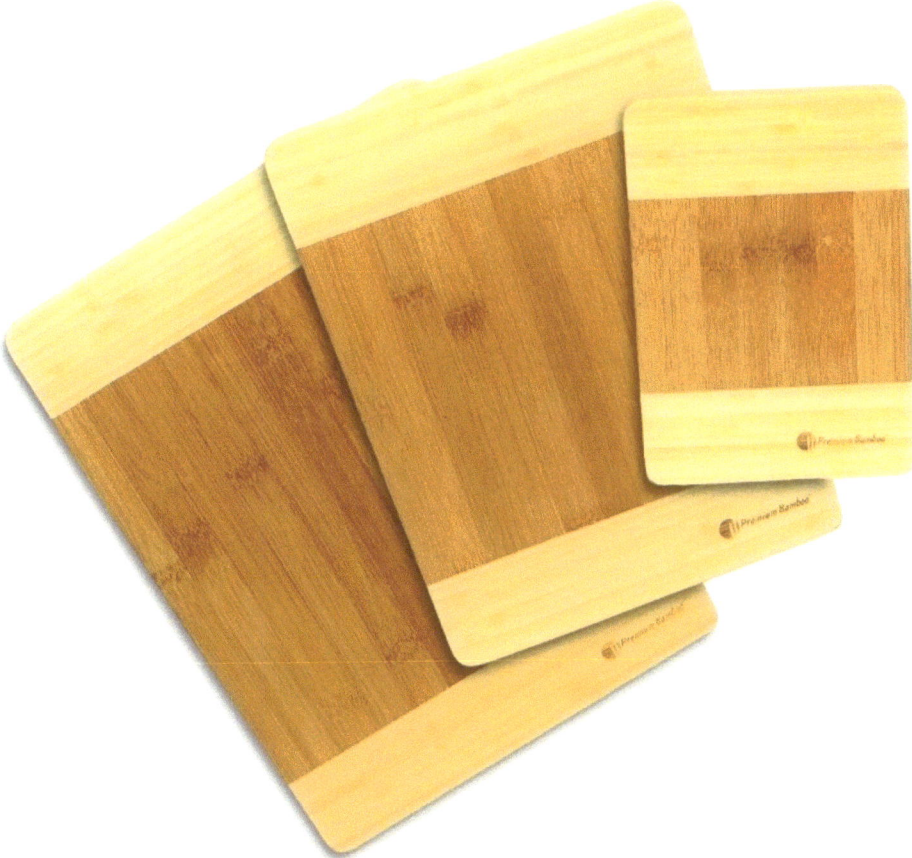

Knife:

Kyocera Revolution Series Paring and Santoku Knife Set

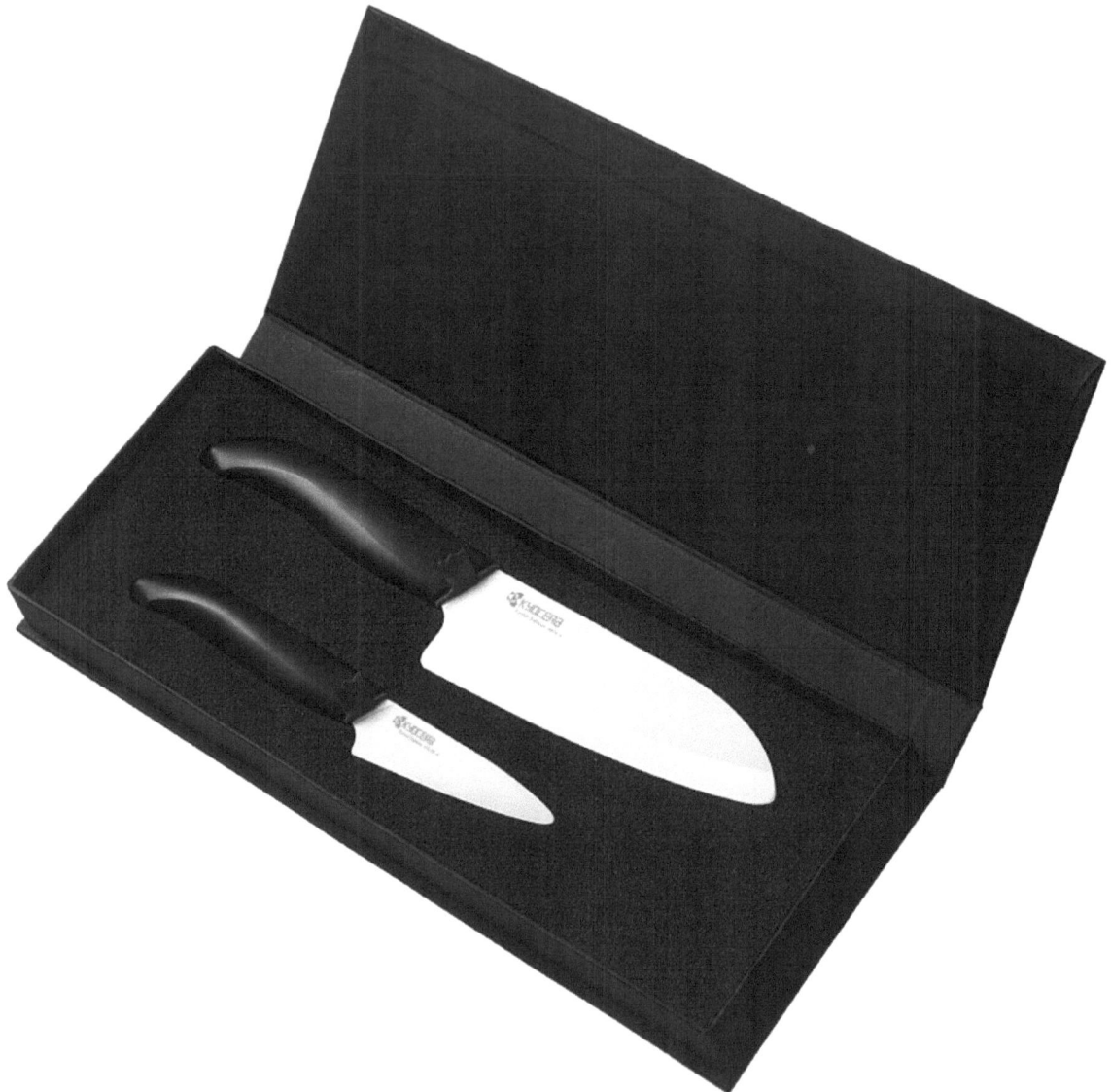

These are some of the items we recommend and personally use however there are many options to chose from. You'll find plenty of other items from our webpage that will make your juice making tasks so much easier to do.

The 3 most important things you'll need will be: **Juicer, Container, and Fruits and Vegetables.**

How much you want to spend on equipment or how fancy a set of knives and glassware you want is totally up to you.

Storage and Shelf Life

Vegetable juice is highly perishable so please drink your juices immediately, or store it properly to retain the optimal nutritional benefits. All juice should be consumed within 24 hours of juicing. It is best to store your juice in a glass jar with an air tight lid, and the juice should be filled to the very top with little to no room for oxygen to avoid the oxidation or damage done to the juice. Melissa personally uses these glasses and they are quite affordable which can be found at your local Crate and Barrel.

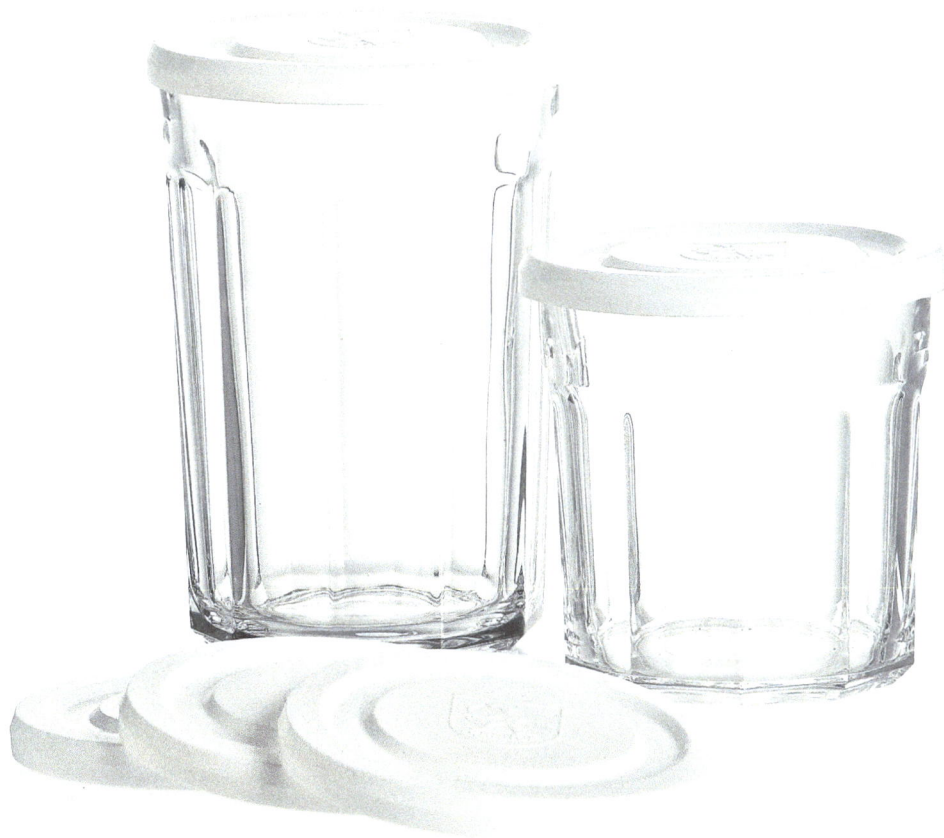

Or online at: <u>Crate and Barrel</u>

Melissa has found them to be very easy to travel with and they do not spill as the lids are air tight.   Jimmy already owns Ball mason jars and they too keep your juice air tight. The important thing to remember is to keep your juice refrigerated and to consume within 24 hours to get the most nutrients from it.

Prepping and Cleaning

An efficient time management routine:

If you have to work during your cleanse, juicing every evening is best to prepare your juices for the next day. That way you can grab your juices in the morning and go. Make 1 juice meal at a time and then store properly, so that you are maximizing the benefits of each juice.

If you are home, or work from home, then juicing each time you are scheduled to consume a glass is ideal. This can be time consuming as you need to clean the juicer once you are finished and don't want to leave the vegetable and fruit waste stuck to your juicer. Most times, you will be able to make 2 or even 3 juices before having to rinse your juicer out, as the leftover fruits and vegetables stuck to the juicer can make it harder to perform. We prefer to make all of our juices in the evening in preparation for the following day for better time management. All juices should be stored in the refrigerator in airtight glass jars with a lid. (See storage and shelf life section)

Please clean your juicer immediately after you have finished juicing . Follow the instruction manual for your particular juicer to get the most life from it.

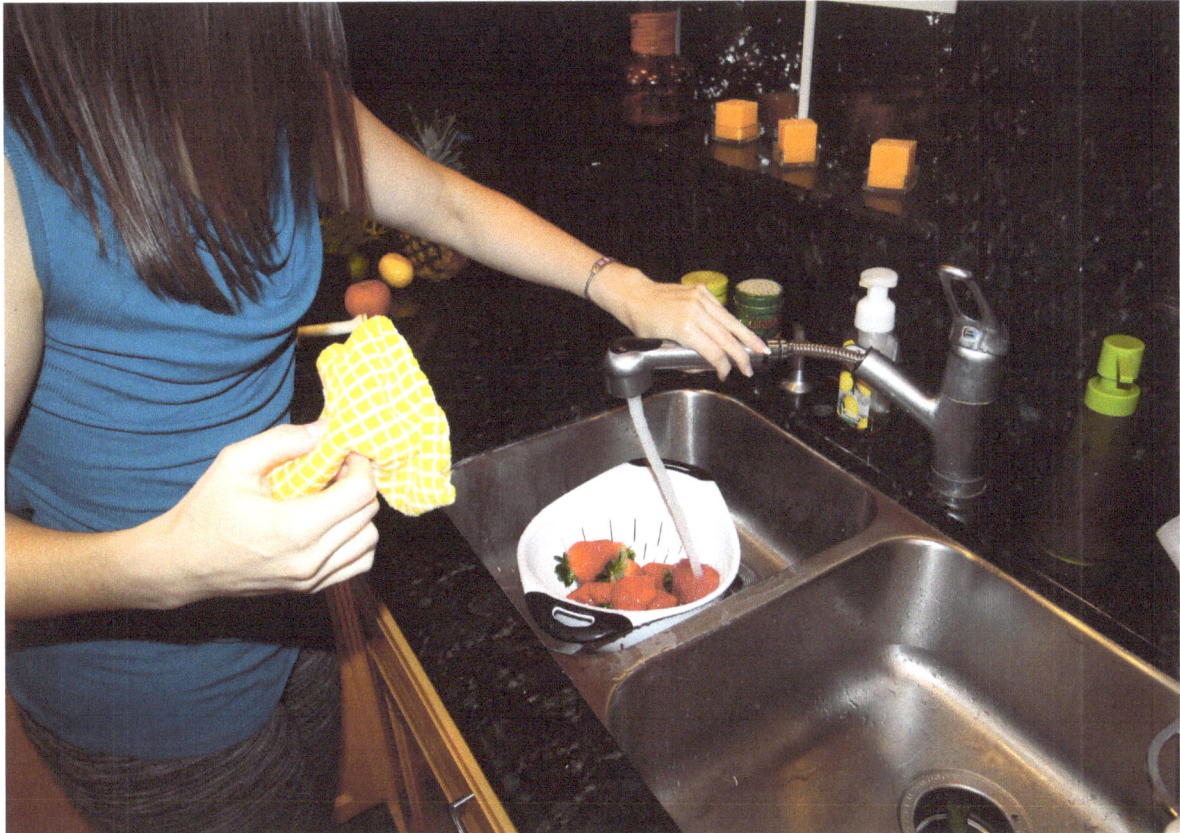

Photo by James Delong

Cleaning and Prepping Tips

•   Rinsing/cleaning your fruits and vegetables under warm water and rubbing or scrubbing with your hands should suffice and remove the dirt that is on your produce. Some people prefer other cleaning methods, such as a vegetable wash spray and veggie brush. Please use whatever works for you, just be sure to clean your produce right before you juice.

•   Green leafy vegetables will not need to be cut before feeding them into your juicer, you can juice the leaves and stems

•   Peel all citrus fruits

- Larger fruits and vegetables will need to be cut into quarters or smaller pieces to fit the mouth of your machine before juicing, such as apples, oranges, and bell peppers. It is ok to juice the core and seeds (remove the hard stems), most juicers can handle this. Please refrain from cutting your produce until right before juicing, because some of the nutrients begin to deplete after you cut them. If you need to prep, then cutting them the night before is ok.

- Pineapples need to have the skin and core removed before juicing

- Fruits and vegetables that have skin such as carrots, apples and cucumbers do not need to be peeled.

- When juicing melons, cut rinds off and scoop out seeds

- Push your green leafy vegetables through the juicer first, followed by harder fruits and veggies to maximize the juice. I (James) would wrap my leafy veggies around other items like cut apples and then place in the chute together.

- Long produce such as celery and cucumbers - cut in half

- Root vegetables such as beets should be cut into quarters and fed through the juicer in small amounts. They are very hard so you want to go easy on your juicer with small pieces at a time.

- Drink the juice immediately or within 24 hours of juicing.

Shopping list for weight loss recipes

Here's all the fruits and vegetables that you will need for your 3 day detox juicing recipes:

12 pears
9 apples
6 cups of strawberries
9 cucumbers
4 bunches of celery (enough for 36 stalks of celery)
6 cups of blueberries
5 red beets
3 bunches of kale (enough for 27 kale leaves)
6 oranges
3 lemons
3 bunches of spinach (enough for 9 handfuls)
6 large tomatoes
3 large broccoli stems
1 small watermelon
cinnamon
coconut water (buy as much as you want to drink throughout cleanse in addition to water)

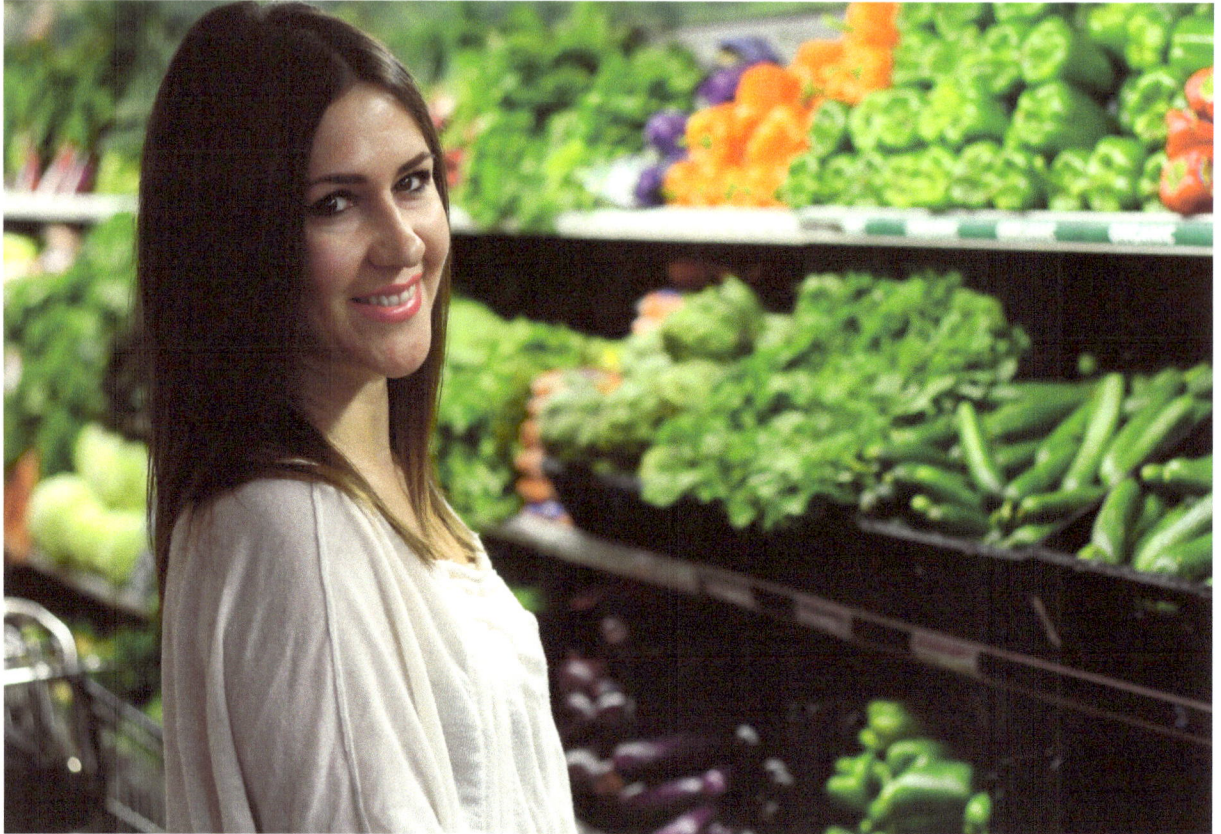

Photo of Melissa buying organic by James Delong

Juicing Recipes for Weight Loss

    A juice cleanse is an effective way to lose weight. Believe it or not, the toxins in your system carry weight too, so as you cleanse your system the pounds can drop off leaving room for a healthier caloric intake. The fruits and vegetables consumed during this cleanse will help alkalize your body, serve as a great liver detoxifier, stabilize blood sugar levels, provide high levels of water intake, increase your metabolism, speed your body's fat burning capacity and fight free radicals in your system.

    Juicing Recipes for Fat Burning:
  **drink coconut water throughout cleanse to boost liver metabolism
  ***for additional weight loss continue this regimen for another cycle (6 days total)

Slim Start

2 Cups of Strawberries
2 Pears
2 Apples

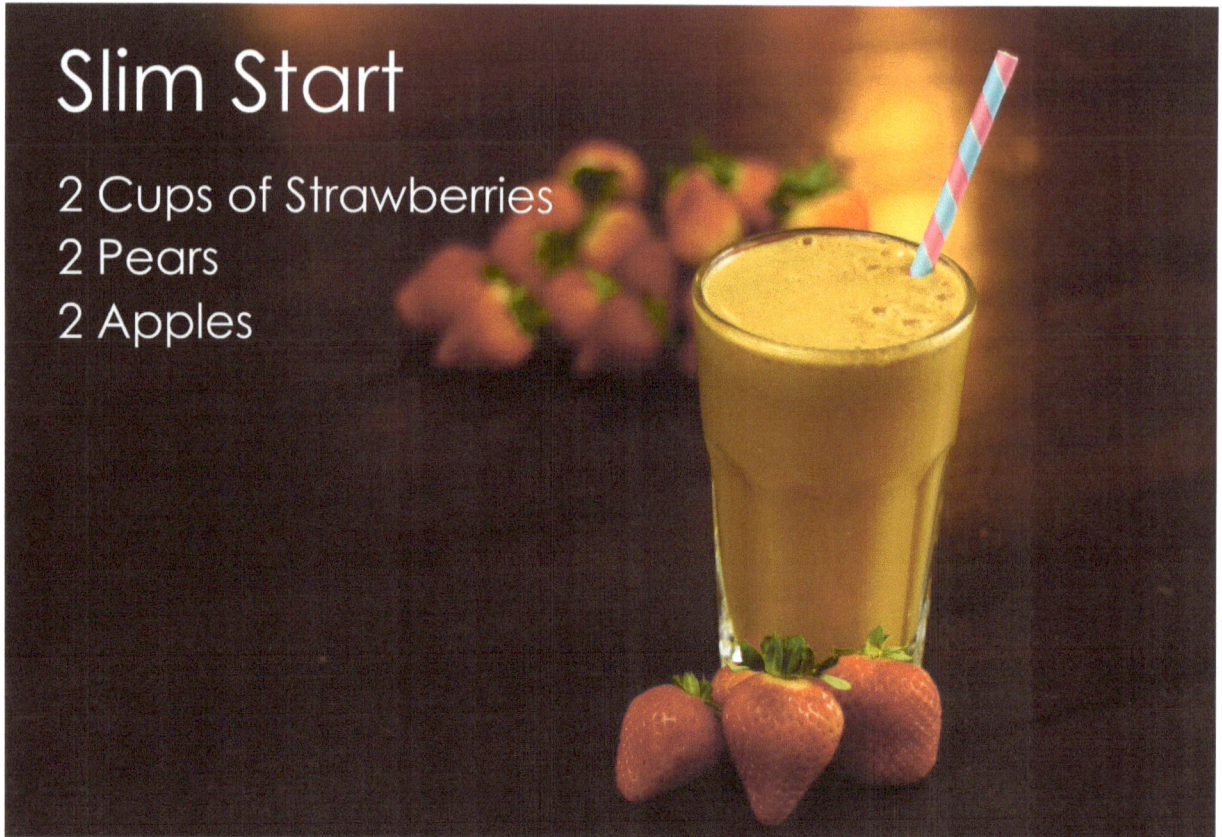

Photo by James Delong

Juice 1: Slim Start

2 pears

2 apples

2 cups of strawberries

Juice 2: Red Reducer

2 medium cucumbers

3 stalks of celery

2 cups of blueberries

½ red beet

Skinnie Minnie

5 Large Kale Leaves
5 Celery Stalks
1 Orange
1 Lemon

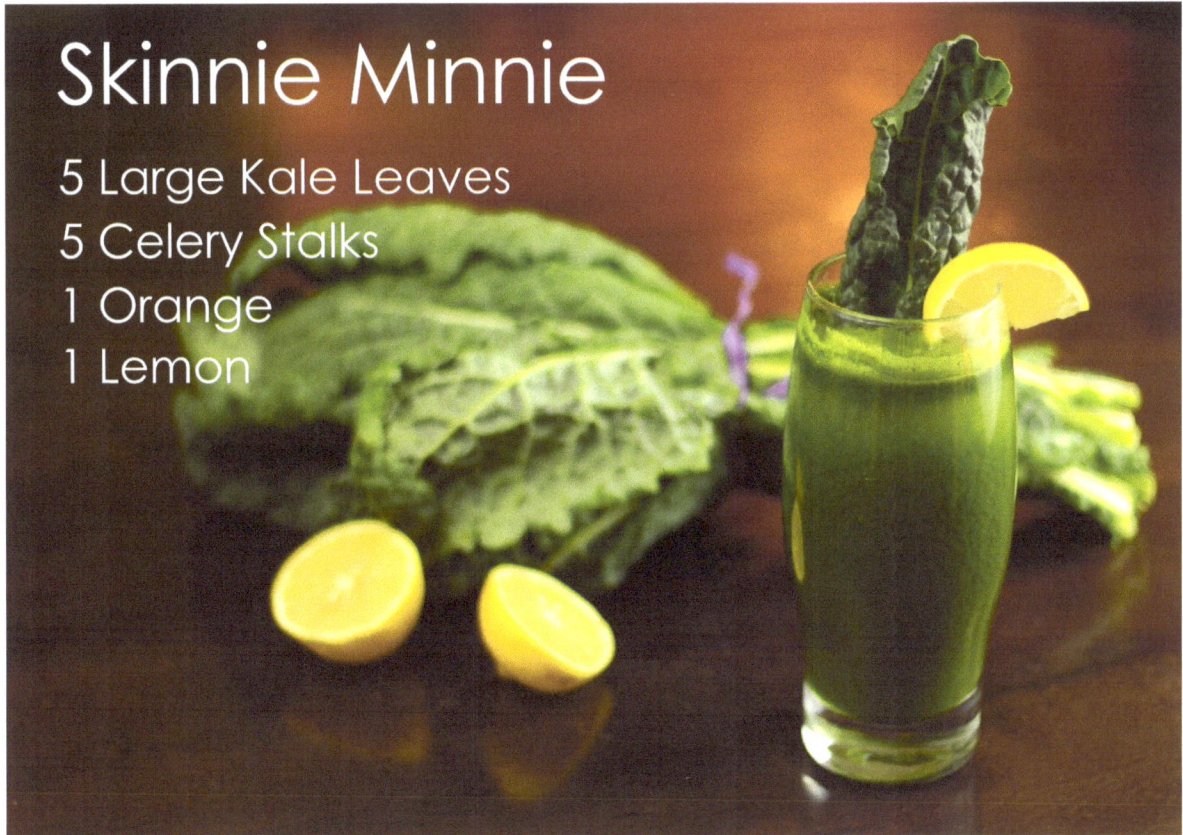

Photo by James Delong

Juice 3: Skinny Minnie

5 large kale leaves

5 stalks of celery

1 large orange

1 lemon, peeled

Juice 4: Bloody Slim

4 large kale leaves

1 red beet

1 large broccoli stem

1 large orange, peeled

Fat Fighter

3 Handfuls of Spinach
2 Large Tomatoes
1 Cucumber
2 Pears

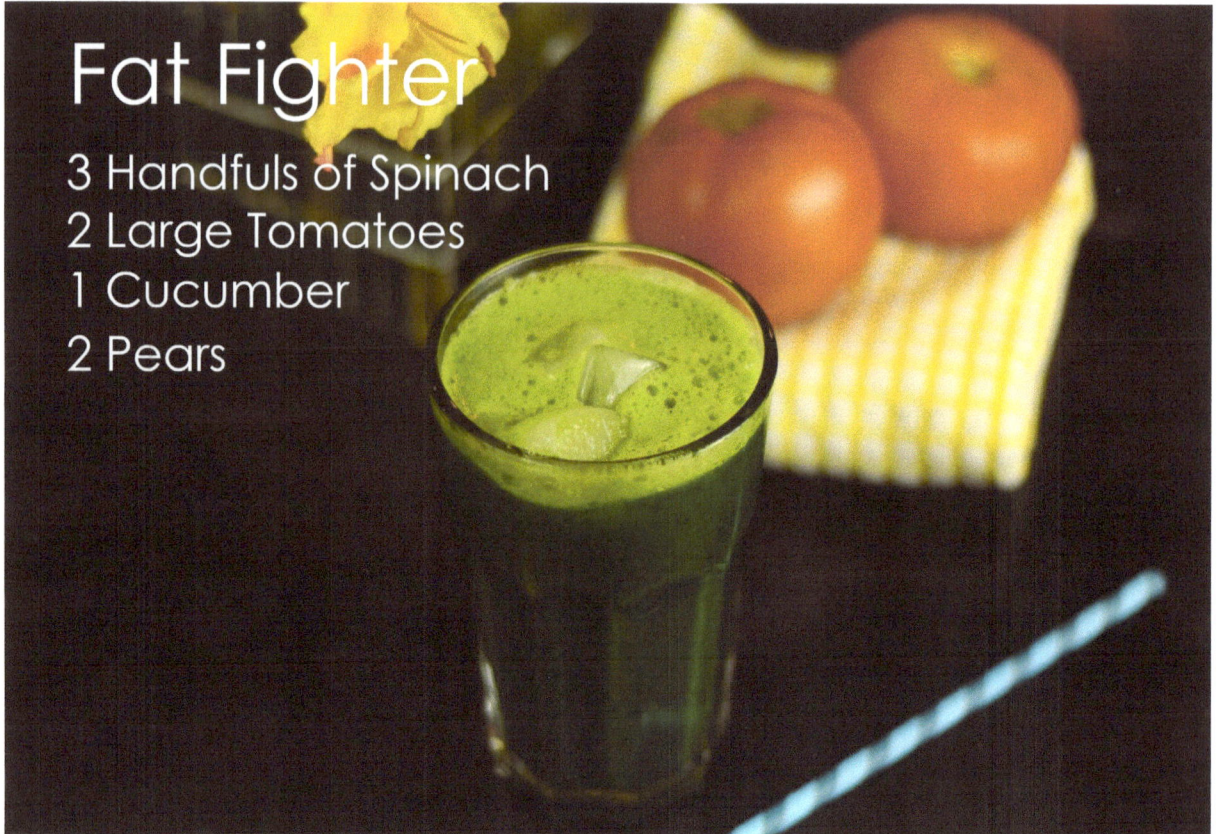

Photo by James Delong

Juice 5: Fat Fighter

3 handfuls of spinach

2 large tomato

1 medium cucumber

2 pears

Juice 6: Late Hydrate

4 celery stalks

1 cup of watermelon

1 large apple

dash of cinnamon

Day 1 - Weight Loss Cleanse

Juicing Schedule

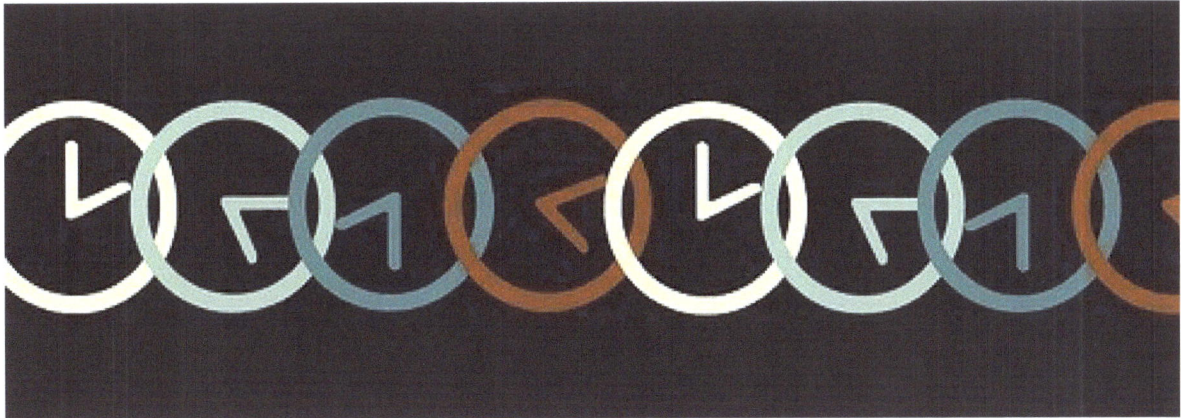

Photo by: Sean MacEntee

Below you will find the juices and schedule that you should adhere to as closely as possible.

Remember to drink lots of water, preferably a gallon a day and if you want to add some variety you can also drink coconut water.

[Each day of Jimmy's 3 day detox he had 32 ounces of coconut water to keep him hydrated along with at least 8 cups of water.]

Here's the schedule:

8am Juice 1: **Slim Start**

10am Juice 2: **Red Reducer**

12pm Juice 3: **Skinny Minnie**

2pm Juice 4: **Bloody Slim**

4pm Juice 5: **Fat Fighter**

6pm Juice 6: **Late Hydrate**

*The schedule above is just an example, you don't have to have a juice at those exact times but the key is to have something roughly every two to three hours.

Today is day 1 of your detox and a very important thing to note here is how you are going to feel if this is your first time.

Some people may feel sick at first which is caused by a Herx Reaction (the technical term is Jarisch-Herxheimer Reaction). **This is the whole 'feeling worse before feeling better' phase.**

While your body detoxifies it's releasing old bacteria, viruses, and toxins back into your body so that it can be totally flushed out. During this time you might feel under the weather, have a headache, or just feel beat. This is common and will pass so let's push through it together.

My (Jimmy) first time detoxifying was years ago when I gave the Master Cleanse (also known as 10 Day Cleanse or The Lemonade Diet) a try. During the evening on the first day I felt somewhat feverish and I can't tell you how the Salt water flush made me feel but let's just say it's an expletive. The first day my stomach was constantly growling and the next day a big time headache was added to the mix.

I consider myself to have somewhat decent Will Power (I stopped drinking alcohol for a year just for the heck of it, so 10 days of something like this can't beat me.) so I continued to day 2 as norm and felt a little off and wasn't sure why. When I got to my third day of detoxifying something happened. I want to let you in on something that changed my life forever. While in bed the second night I had abdominal pains like no ones business and when the morning came I couldn't get up. I thought it was due to the crunches or workout from the days prior. Being I haven't worked out in awhile, I knew I was going to be sore but not like this.

Now this is not to scare you off as the issues I went through had nothing to do with my detox, but on that third day of my cleanse I was cramped up on the couch and couldn't move an inch and that's when I gave in and called my ex. She stopped by to check on me and wanted to have me go to the clinic but I was hard headed and refused to until threatened that she would call my older brother if I don't see a doctor. So after a little bit of me being a pain in the ass she was finally able to rush me to the hospital.

I am so thankful of her (you didn't read that! j/k) for being persistent and getting me to go because from what I was told by the doctor I was extremely lucky because my appendix was about to erupt and things couldn't have gotten real bad.

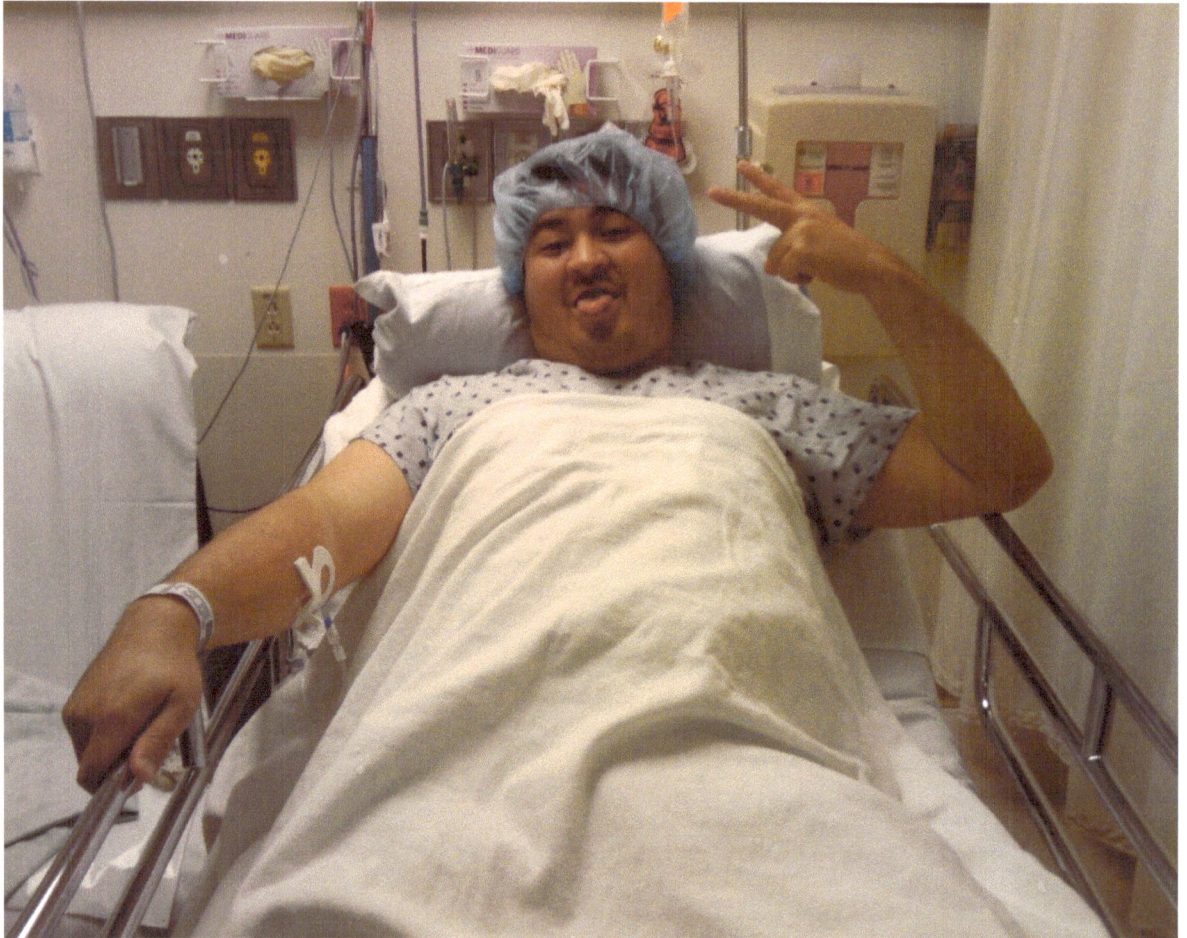
Photo: James Delong

What a bummer because I never did get to finish the Master Cleanse but I was able to make use of the expensive maple syrup that was part of that cleanse's ingredients. Bet your tush I had pancakes after all the stuff I went through and those days I spent cooped up at the hospital.

After all that mess and having a bad experience with the first go round with cleansing I now know what I liked and didn't like about that particular cleansing method.

Moving forward to my most recent 3-day Detox:
I wished I had taken the advice of Melissa to eat healthy meals the week prior to detoxing. I'm 100% certain that it would have eased me more into the

juicing phase and made the hunger pangs more tolerable. Nope, I went cold turkey and while I did have headaches it wasn't that bad.

Some of the side effects that personally happened to me was that I felt colder than usual which is weird for me because I put out major heat. I haven't slept with a blanket in months and the second and third day of detoxing while going to bed I continued to leave the ceiling fan on like normal but had to bundle up because I was freezing.

Second day I also went to bed about two hours earlier than usual and slept the whole night through.

As you can tell from my experience that by knowing what to expect ahead of time it will make your process of entering a detox that much easier to deal with. I don't think what I went through was all that bad as on my fourth day I felt 100% normal and actually had more energy than before.

In fact I even decided to go walking for 30 minutes that night.

One quick note: I did use the restroom 2-3 times more than normal on those those three days. So please be prepared for that while you detox.

Day 2 - Weight Loss Cleanse

Juicing Schedule - Same as previous day

8am Juice 1: **Slim Start**

10am Juice 2: **Red Reducer**

12pm Juice 3: **Skinny Minnie**

2pm Juice 4: **Bloody Slim**

4pm Juice 5: **Fat Fighter**

6pm Juice 6: **Late Hydrate**

As you begin day 2, you will most likely have a headache if you are used to beginning your morning with coffee or tea due to lack of caffeine. Drinking water throughout the day as often as you can should help reduce the severity of those headaches. Remember you can also drink herbal non caffeinated teas throughout the day as well, in addition to coconut water. In fact we encourage it.

Drink your juice as soon as you can in the morning and if the 6 glasses per day aren't enough, feel free to juice more because it won't hurt you. You can repeat one of the recipes above or create your own. Don't feel you are stuck to just these recipes. These however are purposely created for your specific goal.

My (Melissa) first time juicing wasn't as bad as everyone had warned it would be. Before my first cleanse I was already eating clean so my symptoms were barely there at all. I had a minor headache from not being able to drink caffeinated tea (english breakfast is my favorite) but it wasn't anything that slowed me down and drinking water really helped.

The purpose of my cleanse was an effort to clear my skin from an acne flare up. I knew it was possible that something I was putting into my body was causing the inflammation and by day 2, I was really seeing that calm down. By the end of the day my skin had made remarkable progress. Definitely motivation for me to keep going!

I did experience hunger pangs and of course they were worse when I would smell food or would be around someone who was eating. I remember going to the movies with a friend one night and took my juice drinks to the theater. It really helped being prepared no matter where I was because the vegetable and fruit juice does add more of a fuller feeling compared to just water.

Being the fitness junkie that I am, I was even able to go to the gym on day 2 of my cleanse and had an incredible amount of energy on the elliptical. I did a steady pace (no HIIT training) for 20 minutes and my breathing was actually easier than it usually is when I'm consuming solids.

This was my personal experience so it is best to listen to your body, and if you feel fatigued then take the time to relax and don't push it. 1 more day to go!

Day 3 - Weight Loss Cleanse

Juicing Schedule - Same as previous day

8am Juice 1: **Slim Start**

10am Juice 2: **Red Reducer**

12pm Juice 3: **Skinny Minnie**

2pm Juice 4: **Bloody Slim**

4pm Juice 5: **Fat Fighter**

6pm Juice 6: **Late Hydrate**

On the final day of your cleanse, continue to drink plenty of water and coconut water to help combat cravings and any headaches that may be present.

Day 3 can sometimes be the hardest (depending on the state of your health) so no matter how difficult, push through and stick to the schedule. For Jimmy, the first two days was the most difficult for him and you're almost at the finish line. The fact that this detox does so much for your body in only 72 hours is quite amazing.

If you've noticed today a few things have already happened:
1. You should have more energy (Days 1 and 2, Jimmy was beat!)
2. You've actually dropped a few pounds.
3. Your stomach is flatter
4. And most importantly your body has flushed lots of the toxins from your body

Since this is your last day of the cleanse and you already know what to expect, feel free to add an additional glass of juice to your day if this helps you, especially if you're still getting those headaches and hunger pangs.

Don't fret because tomorrow you can begin easing back into whole foods by following our 3 day nutrition plan. Congratulations on completing your cleanse!

How to lose and maintain a healthy weight

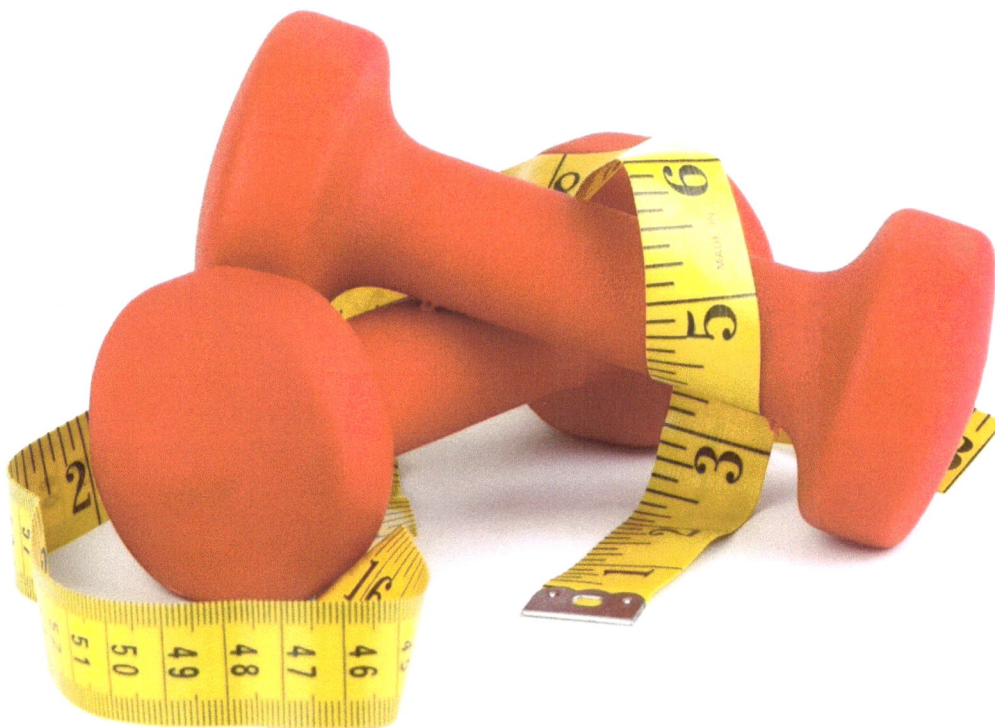

The best and healthiest way to lose weight is to combine healthy eating habits with consistent exercise. This juice cleanse is a great way to start that process, and with any routine change in regards to your health, we always advise that you follow your doctor's orders.

There are many pre-designed weight loss programs available that you can follow. The problem with a majority of them is that they trick you into believing you can still maintain a *healthy* weight while eating processed foods as long as you practice portion control and calorie counting. And while you may drop the necessary weight by doing so, you are trading one problem for another by becoming nutrient deficient when you consume a lot of these processed foods. The term processed isn't limited to just fast food, it also applies to pre-made boxed dinners, particularly diet dinners.

Fad diets will continue to come and go, but the tried and true method to maintaining your health and goal weight will always resort back to including fresh fruits, vegetables, lean meats, healthy fats, beans, nuts and legumes in your diet. The best way to do this is to prepare the food yourself, or be particularly careful when going out to eat. We have found that you can learn a lot about a restaurant just by researching their menu online before you even agree to eat there. Scope the menu and decide before going what you are ok with eating, and what you need to stay away from. Unfortunately many restaurants use pre-frozen processed foods to cut back on prep time when preparing your meals. These frozen processed foods may taste amazing but they are usually loaded with GMO's (genetically modified organism), cancer causing preservatives and other weight gaining properties. **Just one of these meals per week can set you back tremendously** if you are trying to lose weight. You can always ask the waitress or waiter if the food is pre-frozen and they are usually honest when answering.

Start slow when changing your habits; if you like to swing by your favorite fast food place for breakfast every day, then start by eliminating that one habit per week, and work your way up from there. You'll find that eliminating one bad habit at a time *slowly*, rather than going full speed and eliminating all at once, will be much easier to maintain. Before you know it you will have eliminated many of your bad eating habits after a few months. Patience is key when losing weight the natural and healthiest way. It takes your body time to adjust to your new and healthy way of living, so give it time.

One of the best ways to change a bad habit is by replacing it with good one. Replace one unhealthy snack with a juice. It's better for you and you have control of what's in it.

To give you an idea about the types of foods that you should be gravitating toward, we have developed a 3 day Bonus Meal Plan that is included with this juice cleanse. The meal plan includes all whole natural foods that will help speed metabolism, burn fat, build lean muscle, and feed your body with the much needed nutrients needed to survive.

You'll find that you do not need to calorie count as much when you are eating food the way nature intended - food that is minimally processed, food purchased in its most natural form.

Another great benefit of eating whole natural foods is that you will no longer need to kill yourself in the gym in order to maintain a healthy goal weight. You are better off exercising for 20-30 minutes each day rather than 1-2 hours, 2 or 3 days a week. Consistency is key when it comes to nutrition and working out.

We wish you luck on your journey and encourage you to keep in touch with us for more helpful tips and support! We'd love to hear about or see your weight loss progress, so please tweet, comment, or email us with an update! - You can find us at www.juicefam.com

3 Day Nutrition Plan after Detox (Bonus #1)

As a reward for completing your cleanse and to show our appreciation, we have created a 3 day nutritional plan to follow to ease you back into consuming whole foods. This meal plan is free of wheat, gluten, soy and preservatives.

Please drink plenty of water with this meal plan and avoid diet drinks, processed fruit drinks and sodas.

Shopping list:
1 package of steel cut oats
1 carton of rice or almond milk
Brown sugar
Sliced almonds
Herbal tea of choice
3 cups of blueberries
3 cups of organic plain yogurt
3 boneless skinless chicken breasts
3 avocados
Olive oil or vinaigrette dressing of your choice
1 bunch of fresh romaine lettuce, or 2 containers of freshly prepared salad greens
1 pound of sliced organic turkey meat
2 small cucumbers
1 small container of hummus
6 filets of fresh fish or wild caught frozen fish (your choice - cod, halibut, etc)
3 yams or sweet potatoes
1 large bunch of fresh broccoli

Breakfast: *Approx. 305 calories*
Steel cut oatmeal - add rice or almond milk, 1 teaspoon of organic brown sugar and sliced almonds
Herbal tea or freshly pressed fruit juice
Follow cooking instructions on carton of oatmeal. Add remaining ingredients

once finished cooking.

Mid morning snack: *Approx. 230 calories if choosing whole milk yogurt*
1 cup of fresh blueberries with 1 cup of organic plain yogurt
Mix and enjoy

Lunch: *Approx. 700 calories (knock off 300 calories by removing avocado)*
1 Grilled chicken breast (sliced) served over a greens salad, topped with sliced avocado and preferably olive oil. If you prefer a tastier dressing, you can add vinaigrette (avoid heavy cream based dressings).

Afternoon snack: *Approx. 350 calories*
Turkey/hummus/cucumber rollups: (make 3 or 4 rollups)
Spread hummus over a slice of fresh roasted turkey from your local deli, add thinly sliced cucumbers, roll and enjoy!

Dinner: *Approx.* 540 calories if choosing chicken. *Approx.* 480 calories if choosing 2 fish filets.
Leftover grilled chicken from lunch, or grilled fish of choice. Baked yam or sweet potato, steamed broccoli.
Feel free to season with fresh butter (no margarine) and a small amount of sea salt or Himalayan salt

Acne Cleanse and Healthier Skin Shopping List

Shopping list for Acne recipes: (please reference our list of organically preferred foods in our Why Organic section)

Here's all the fruits and vegetables that you will need for your 3 day detox juicing recipes:

3 oranges

5 lemons

6 green apples

6 red apples

2 bunches of collard greens (enough for 12 collard green leaves)

9 cucumbers

3 green bell peppers

6 yellow bell peppers

2 bunches of green grapes (enough for 6 big handfuls)

3 bunches of kale (enough for 24 kale leaves)

15 carrots

6 cups of blackberries

6 tomatoes

3 large broccoli stems

2 red beets

3 pineapples

2 bunches of spinach (enough for 6 handfuls)

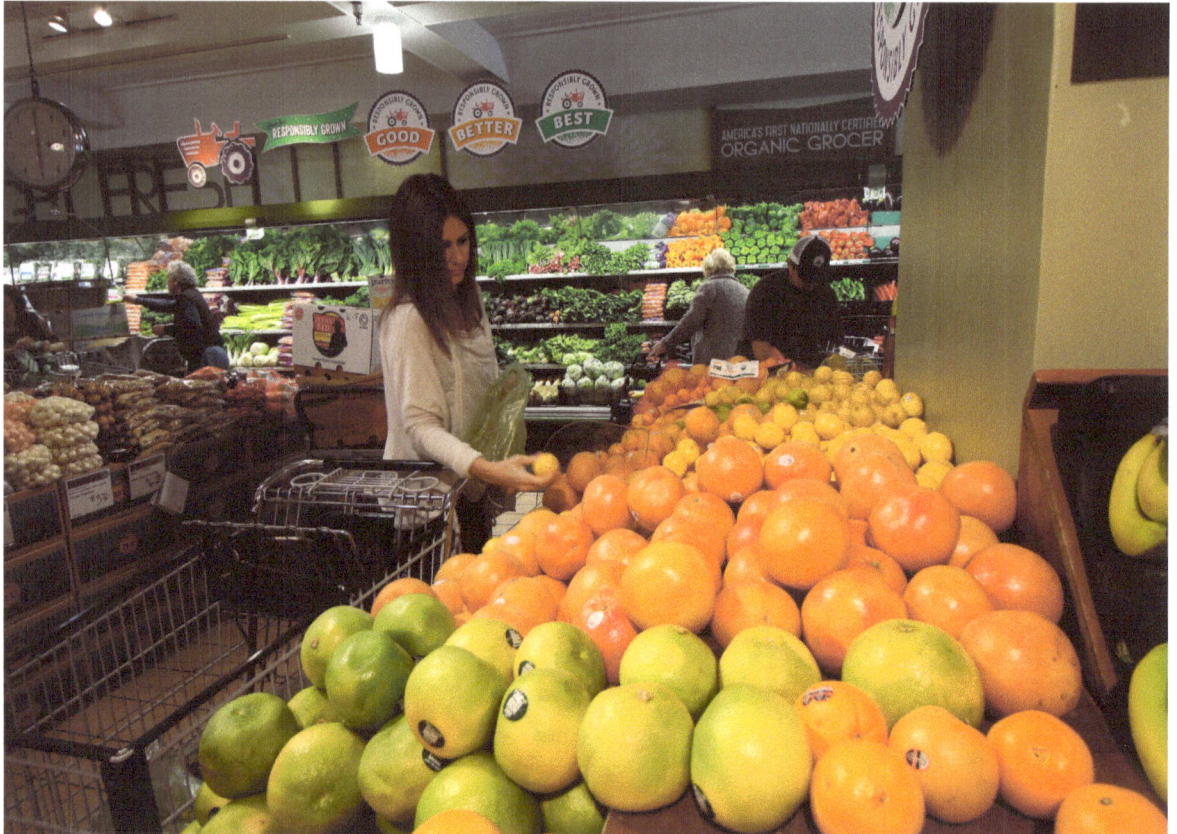

Photo of Melissa buying organic by James Delong

Juicing Recipes for Acne Cleanse and Healthier Skin

A proven way to heal your acne is to start with the inside and get to the source of the problem. These recipes have been carefully designed to target problem areas and reduce irritation. The benefits received from this cleanse will strengthen cell walls to prevent from scarring, provide bioflavonoids which are a natural anti-inflammatory, are rich in vitamins A, B complex, C, E, K, beta carotene, antioxidants and fight radical damage. All of which equals clearer healthier skin.

Acne cleanse - Juicing recipes:

* Helpful note - These juices may be more refreshing served over ice

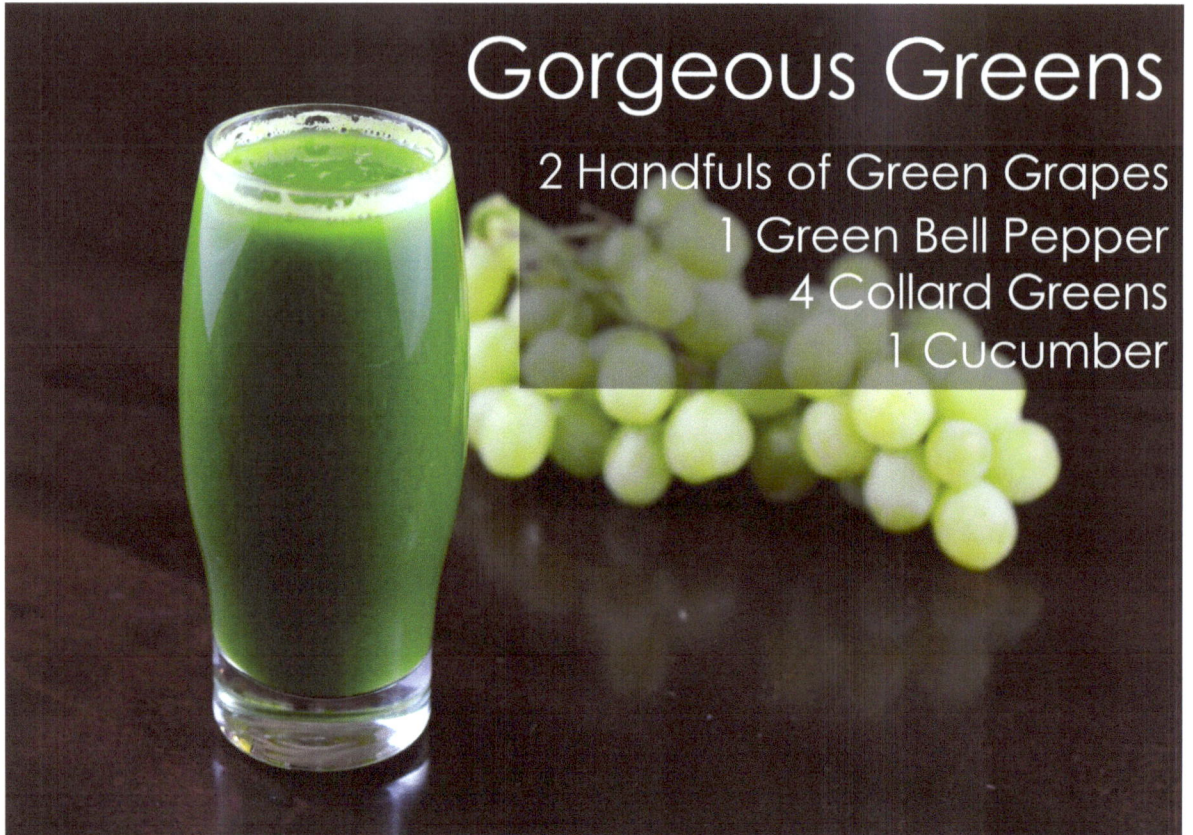

Gorgeous Greens

2 Handfuls of Green Grapes
1 Green Bell Pepper
4 Collard Greens
1 Cucumber

Photo by James Delong

Juice 1: Cool Citrus Riser

1 large orange, peeled
1 lemon, peeled
2 green apples

Juice 2: Gorgeous Greens

4 large collard green leaves
1 medium cucumber
1 green bell pepper
2 big handfuls of green grapes

Bloody Good Skin

1 Large Broccoli Stem
2 Tomatoes
1/2 Red Beet
1/2 Cucumber
2 Red Apples

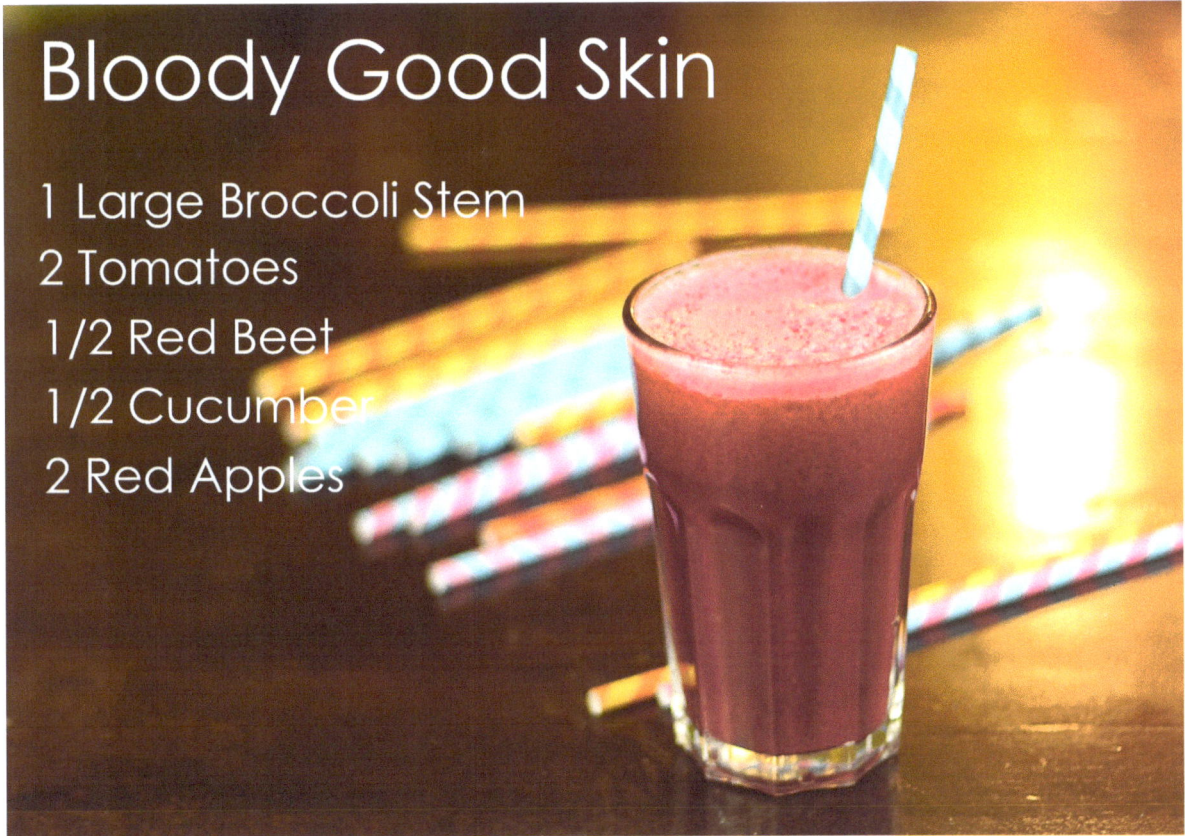

Photo by James Delong

Juice 3: Deep Crush

5 large kale leaves

5 carrots

2 cups of blackberries

Juice 4: Bloody Good Skin

2 tomatoes

1 large broccoli stem

½ red beet

½ cucumber

2 red apples

Crystal Clear

2 Yellow Bell Peppers
1/2 Cucumber
1/2 Lemon
1/2 Pineapple

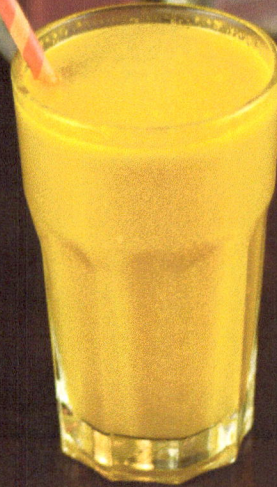

Photo by James Delong

Juice 5: Crystal Clear

2 yellow bell peppers

½ cucumber

½ lemon peeled

½ of a pineapple (skin cut off, and cored)

Juice 6: Emerald Twilight

2 handfuls of spinach

3 large kale leaves

1 medium cucumber

½ of a pineapple (skin cut off, and cored

Day 1 - Acne Cleanse

Juicing Schedule

Below you will find the juices and schedule that you should adhere to as closely as possible.
Remember to drink lots of water, preferably a gallon a day and if you want to add some variety you can also drink coconut water.

Here's the schedule:

8am Juice 1: **Cool Citrus Riser**

10am Juice 2: **Gorgeous Greens**

12pm Juice 3: **Deep Crush**

2pm Juice 4: **Bloody Good Skin**

4pm Juice 5: **Crystal Clear**

6pm Juice 6: **Emerald Twilight**

*The schedule above is just an example, you don't have to have a juice at those exact times but the key is to have something roughly every two to three hours.

Day 2 - Acne Cleanse

Juicing Schedule - Same as previous day

8am Juice 1: **Cool Citrus Riser**

10am Juice 2: **Gorgeous Greens**

12pm Juice 3: **Deep Crush**

2pm Juice 4: **Bloody Good Skin**

4pm Juice 5: **Crystal Clear**

6pm Juice 6: **Emerald Twilight**

One more day left, you can do it.

Day 3 - Acne Cleanse

Juicing Schedule - Same as previous day

8am Juice 1: **Cool Citrus Riser**

10am Juice 2: **Gorgeous Greens**

12pm Juice 3: **Deep Crush**

2pm Juice 4: **Bloody Good Skin**

4pm Juice 5: **Crystal Clear**

6pm Juice 6: **Emerald Twilight**

On the final day of your cleanse, continue to drink plenty of water and coconut water to help combat cravings and any headaches that may be present.

Congratulations on completing your Healthier Skin cleanse!

Just like the weight loss cleanse we want to go above and beyond and also provide you with another 3 day Bonus Meal Plan that was designed to use after this particular detox.

Preventing and minimizing acne from within

As I'm sure you are learning by now, a lot of ailments can be healed internally through proper nutrition and whole natural foods without the use of pharmaceutical drugs. The ingredients chosen for this cleanse were pulled from a list of vegetables and fruits that are specifically beneficial in fighting acne, and we have listed that below for a better understanding of how this can benefit you.

To assist you with meeting your goal of reducing and removing acne completely we encourage you to rotate the below foods in your diet. While this probably won't fix your issue overnight, it most certainly will pay off over time, and placing your focus on what is beneficial for you in addition to completing a cleanse as often as you are able to, will only have positive effects on your health and your skin.

As an added bonus we have designed a 3 day meal plan that you can follow after your cleanse, because this meal plan was also specifically created with foods that fight acne and promote healthy skin. We hope that you use the meal plan along with the information below as a starting point for healthier food choices!

Foods that are beneficial for fighting acne:

GRAPES: Seeds and fruit contain powerful antioxidants for treating inflammation	BROCCOLI: Vitamins A, B complex, C, and K - antioxidants fight radical damage	CARROTS, BELL PEPPERS, BEETS: Beta carotene which converts to Vitamin A

ORANGES, TOMATOES, MELONS: Vitamin C, Strengthens cells walls to protect from scarring, and bioflavonoids are a natural anti-inflammatory	BLUEBERRIES, RASPBERRIES, BLACKBERRIES, SPINACH, KALE: Strong antioxidants	GRAPEFRUIT, PINEAPPLE, LEMON: Rich in Vitamin C
FISH: Essential fatty acids (omega 3 and omega 6), reduces inflammation	NUTS: Selenium, vitamin E, magnesium, manganese, potassium, calcium and iron	AVOCADO: Rich in vitamin E, can increase skin's vitality
GARLIC: Fights inflammation	SWEET POTATOES: Beta carotene, vitamin C	OATS: Good source of zinc, low in iodine. Zinc can reduce inflammation and kill bacteria
LEAFY GREENS: Rich in vitamin E	APPLES: Pectin and antioxidants	PAPAYAS: Vitamin A and enzymes
CUCUMBERS: Silicon and sulfur	ARTICHOKE: Antioxidants and vitamin C	BROWN RICE: Vitamin B, helps regulate hormones
DANDELION GREENS: One of the best sources of beta carotene	ROMAINE LETTUCE: High chromium content (can stabilize blood sugar	

3 Day Nutrition Plan after Acne Cleanse (Bonus #2)

As a reward for completing your cleanse and to show our appreciation, we have created a 3 day nutritional plan to follow to ease you back into consuming whole foods. This meal plan is free of wheat, gluten, soy and preservatives, it also includes foods that are beneficial for having clear, healthy skin.

Please drink plenty of water with this meal plan and avoid diet drinks, processed fruit drinks and sodas.

Shopping list:

1 cup of blueberries
1 carton of rice or almond milk
Green tea
3 avocados
4 tomatoes
1 package of almond meal
Eggs
Vinaigrette dressing of your choice
1 bunch of fresh romaine lettuce, or 2 containers of freshly prepared salad greens
1 pound of organic ground turkey
2 small cucumbers
Honey or favorite syrup
6 filets of fresh fish or wild caught frozen fish (your choice - cod, halibut, etc)
3 yams or sweet potatoes
1 large bunch of fresh broccoli
1 medium onion
1 bunch of Swiss chard
3 bananas
3 apples
3 jalapeños
Smoked paprika
Cumin
Coriander

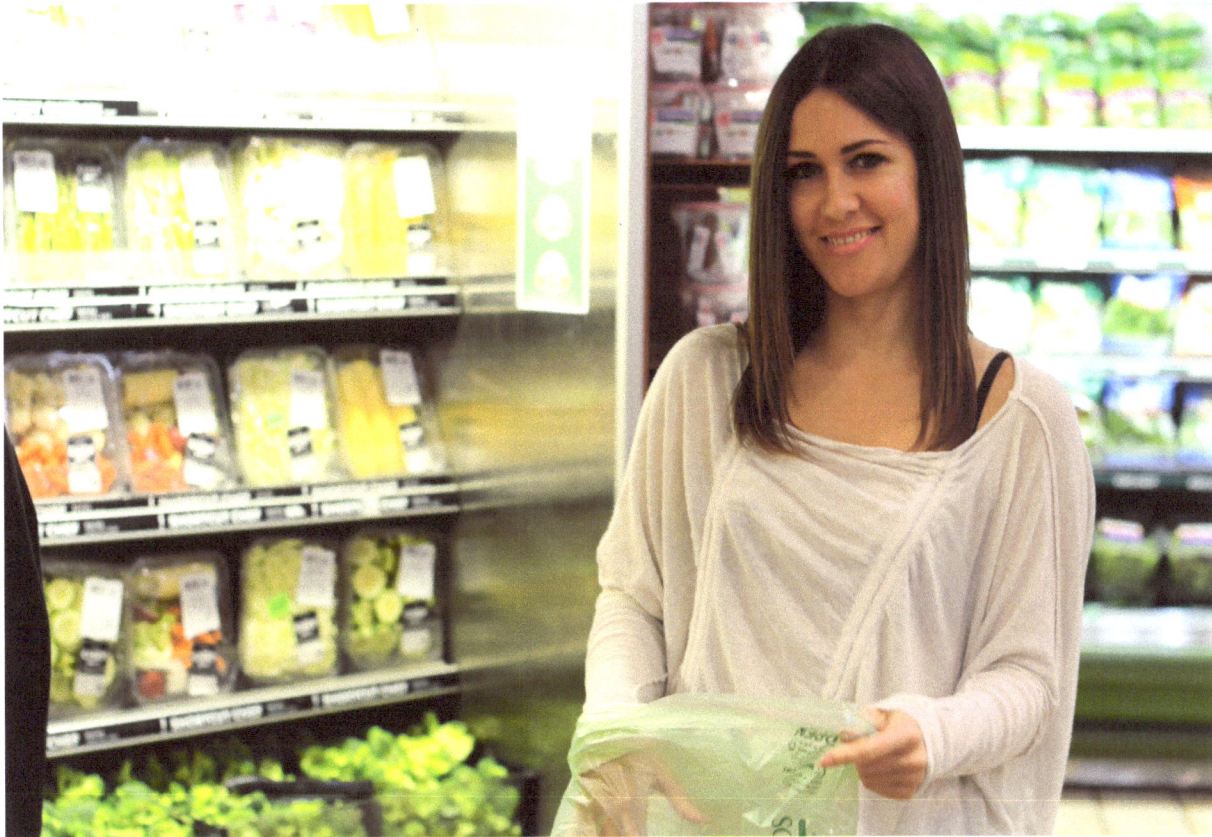

Photo of Melissa buying organic by James Delong

Breakfast: *Approx. 300-400 calories per serving (3 servings per batch)*
Blueberry Breakfast Bake - take 1 cup of almond meal, 1 organic egg, ¼ cup of water, dash of salt and ¾ cup of blueberries. Mix and bake at 350 degrees for 30 minutes. Divide into servings of 3 and use 1 serving for breakfast per day. Drizzle with honey or your favorite syrup.
Green Tea or freshly pressed fruit juice

Mid morning snack: *Approx. 300 calories*
Sliced avocado and tomato

Lunch: *Approx. 300 calories per serving (makes 3-4 servings)*
Turkey taco meat with a side salad - sauté 1 medium onion in 2 tablespoons of canola or coconut oil, add 1 pound of ground turkey, 1 diced jalapeño, 1 diced tomato, 1 tablespoon of smoked paprika, 1 tablespoon of cumin, 1 tablespoon of coriander, salt to taste and ¼ cup of water. Pan cook on medium-low until browned and veggies are soft. Adjust seasonings to taste and add more water if needed.

Serve with a mixed greens salad (romaine, kale, dandelion greens, whichever you prefer), topped with cucumber and your favorite vinaigrette (avoid cream based dressings).

Afternoon snack: *Approx. 350 calories*
Blended smoothie - Combine 1 Swiss chard leaf, 1 banana, 1 apple with 1 cup of rice milk. Blend and enjoy

Dinner: *Approx.* 300 calories if having leftover lunch. *Approx.* 480 calories if choosing 2 fish filets.
Leftover lunch, or 2 grilled fish fillets of choice with baked yam or sweet potato, steamed broccoli.
Feel free to season with fresh butter (no margarine) and a small amount of sea salt or Himalayan salt

Energy Boost Shopping List

Shopping list for Energy:

Here's all the fruits and vegetables that you will need for your 3 day detox juicing recipes:

- 12 cups of strawberries
- 9 large oranges
- 6 lemons
- 9 1 inch pieces of ginger
- 3 bunches of kale (enough for 24 kale leaves)
- 9 cucumbers
- 6 large broccoli stems
- 2 bunches of Swiss chard (enough for 9 Swiss chard leaves)
- 9 carrots
- 9 tomatoes
- 6 red beets
- 3 cups of blackberries
- 2 bunches of spinach (enough for 6 handfuls)
- 5 bunches of arugula (enough for 9 handfuls)
- 1 bunch of collard green leaves (enough for 6 leaves)
- 9 tangerines
- 1 pineapple

Juicing Recipes for Energy Boost and Focus

One of the best ways to sustain energy is to fuel properly by consuming foods that do not weigh you down. It can be easy to consume heavy starch and fatty foods over time, which is why a cleanse is a great way to strip those energy suckers from your body.

The benefits received from this cleanse will assist with energy circulation, regulate energy levels, supply glucose to your blood, as well as provide iron, vitamins A, B, C, and K, boost serotonin levels and improve your mood.

Juicing Recipes for Energy and Focus
**drink coconut water throughout this cleanse to boost energy

Muscle Might

5 Kale Leaves
1 Cucumber
1 Broccoli Stem
1 Orange
1 Ginger

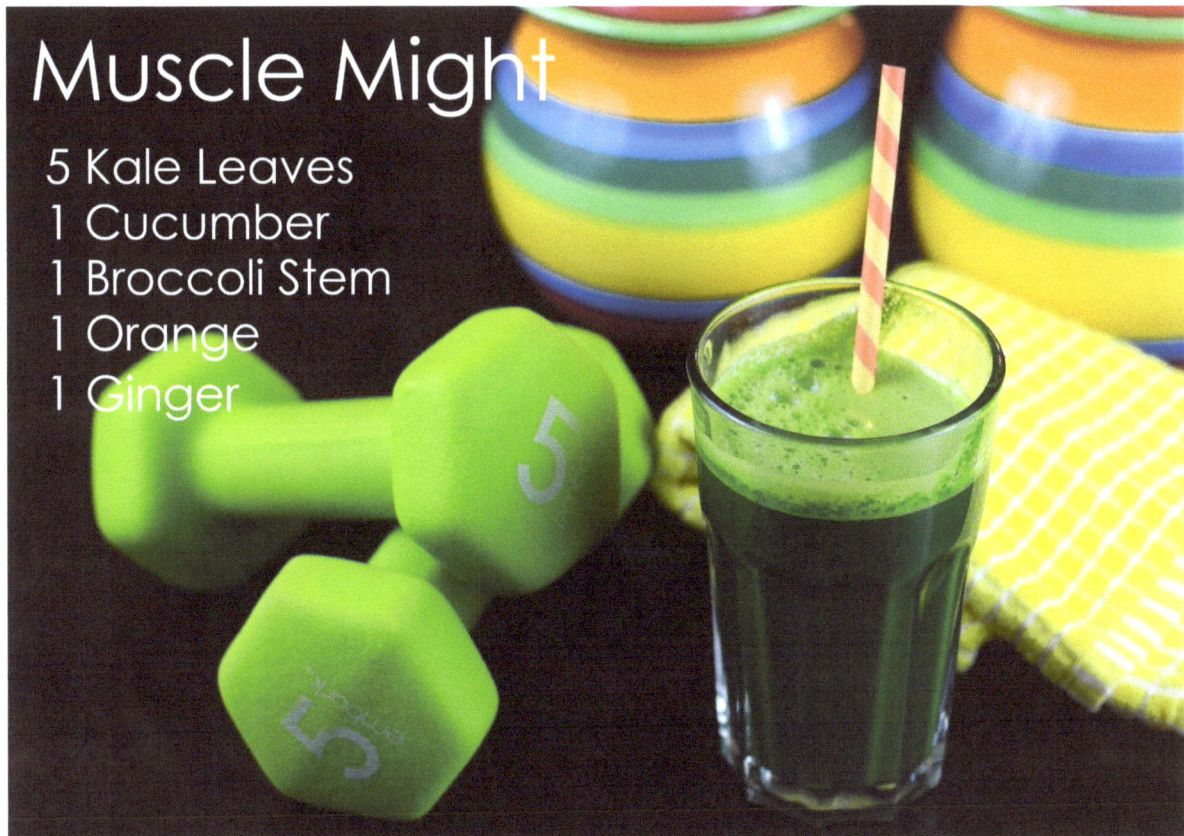

Photo by James Delong

Juice 1: Sunrise Sip

2 cups of strawberries

2 large oranges, peeled

1 lemon, peeled

1 inch piece of ginger

Juice 2: Muscle Might

5 large kale leaves

1 medium cucumber

1 large broccoli stem

1 large orange

1 inch piece of ginger

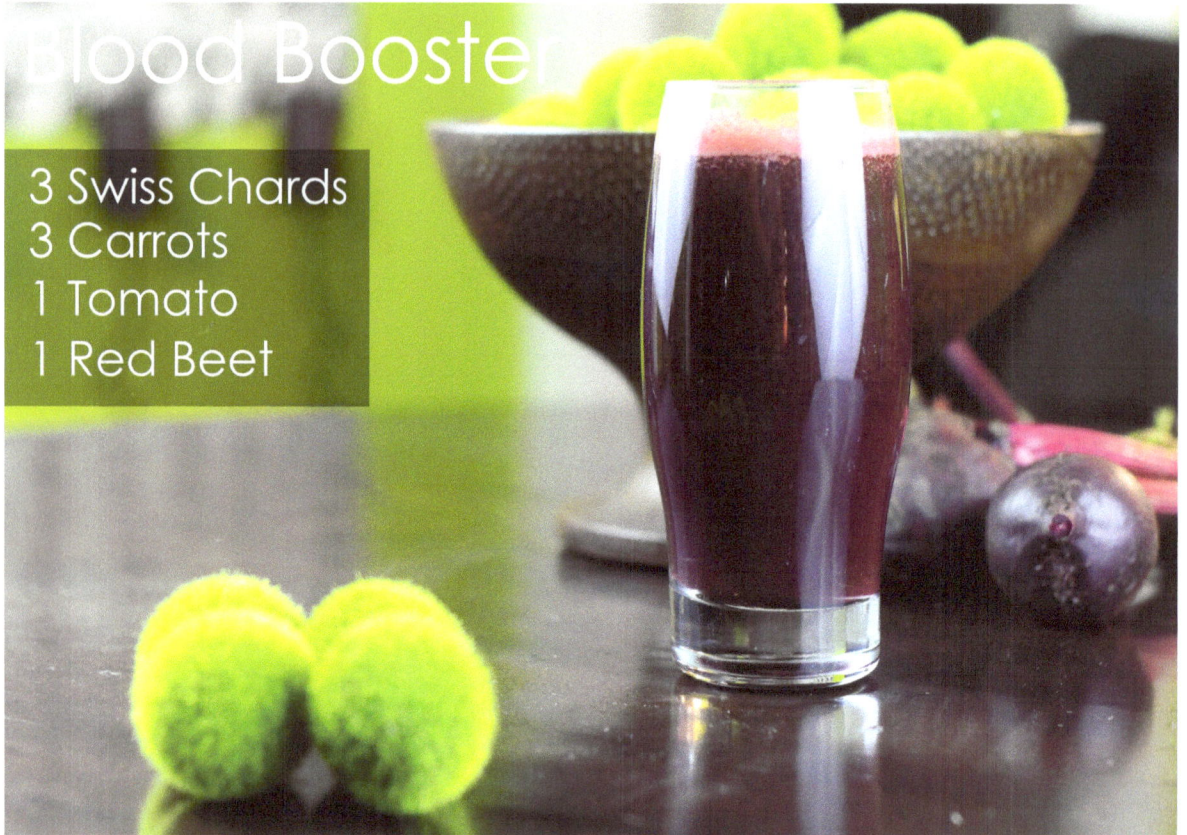

Blood Booster

3 Swiss Chards
3 Carrots
1 Tomato
1 Red Beet

Photo by James Delong

Juice 3: Blood Booster

3 large Swiss chard leaves

3 large carrots

1 large tomato

1 red beet

1 cup of blackberries

1 lemon, peeled

Juice 4: Berry Blush

2 handfuls of spinach

1 medium cucumber

1 red beet

2 cups of strawberries

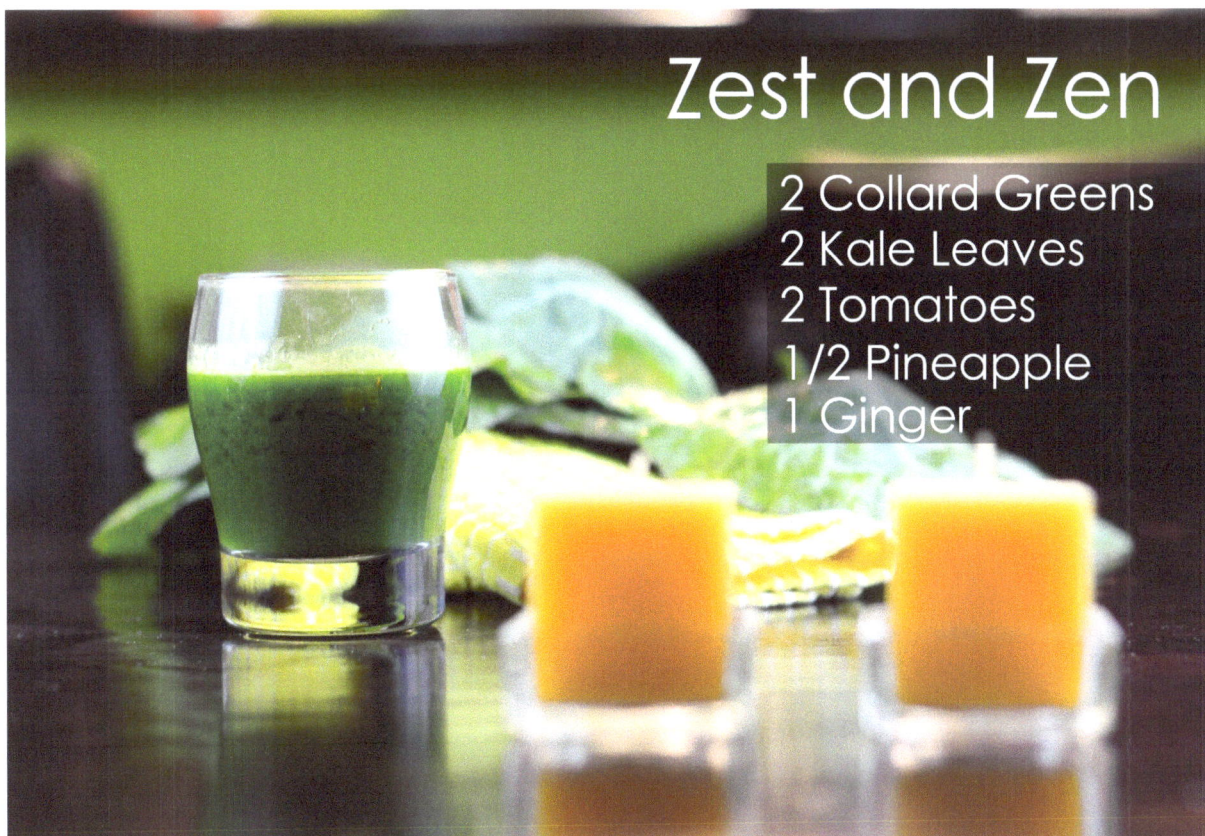

Zest and Zen

2 Collard Greens
2 Kale Leaves
2 Tomatoes
1/2 Pineapple
1 Ginger

Photo by James Delong

Juice 5: Vita-C Energy

3 large handfuls of arugula

1 large broccoli stem

1 medium cucumber

3 tangerines

Juice 6: Zest and Zen

2 large collard green leaves

3 large kale leaves

2 tomatoes

⅓ of a pineapple, skin removed and cored

1 inch piece of ginger

Day 1 - Energy Boost and Focus Cleanse

Juicing Schedule

Below you will find the juices and schedule that you should adhere to as closely as possible.
Remember to drink lots of water, preferably a gallon a day and if you want to add some variety you can also drink coconut water.

Here's the schedule:

8am Juice 1: **Sunrise Sip**

10am Juice 2: **Muscle Might**

12pm Juice 3: **Blood Booster**

2pm Juice 4: **Berry Blush**

4pm Juice 5: **Vita-C Energy**

6pm Juice 6: **Zest and Zen**

*The schedule above is just an example, you don't have to have a juice at those exact times but the key is to have something roughly every two to three hours.

Day 2 - Energy Boost and Focus Cleanse

Juicing Schedule - Same as previous day

Here's the schedule:

8am Juice 1: **Sunrise Sip**

10am Juice 2: **Muscle Might**

12pm Juice 3: **Blood Booster**

2pm Juice 4: **Berry Blush**

4pm Juice 5: **Vita-C Energy**

6pm Juice 6: **Zest and Zen**

One more day left, you can do it.

Day 3 - Energy Boost and Focus Cleanse

Juicing Schedule - Same as previous day

Here's the schedule:

8am Juice 1: **Sunrise Sip**

10am Juice 2: **Muscle Might**

12pm Juice 3: **Blood Booster**

2pm Juice 4: **Berry Blush**

4pm Juice 5: **Vita-C Energy**

6pm Juice 6: **Zest and Zen**

On the final day of your cleanse, continue to drink plenty of water and coconut water to help combat cravings and any headaches that may be present.

Helpful Tips For Maintaining Better Energy

Now that you've completed your 3 day detox, we want to provide some helpful tips on maintaining your energy throughout each day. With a few minor adjustments, you can avoid the afternoon lull that so many of us experience shortly after we eat lunch.

Drink plenty of water:
Mild hydration can cause your blood to thicken which requires your heart to pump harder, resulting in fatigue. Water is the best source for hydration compared to energy drinks, caffeine and other beverages loaded with sugar.

Eat breakfast:
Eating a healthy breakfast is a great way to set the tone for the day. It activates your metabolism and maintains your blood sugar levels so that they don't crash and leave you feeling lethargic. Starting with a healthy protein such as organic eggs, oatmeal or a healthy protein drink, can provide fuel to hold you over until lunch.

Eat small meals throughout the day:
Choosing your foods wisely, coupled with eating smaller meals often throughout the day can do wonders for your energy. Backing off of refined carbs and sugars, and increasing lean proteins, healthy fats and vegetables can maintain healthy blood sugar levels in addition to satisfying your hunger longer, resulting in less energy spikes and lulls.

Avoid sodas and energy drinks:
Processing large amounts of sugar can cause your body to work extra hard, resulting in an energy crash.

Exercise consistently:
Consistent exercise releases endorphins which improve your mood, in addition to getting your blood pumping which provides an energy boost.

Additional Helpful Tips

Helpful tips about fruits and vegetables when juicing

We get asked a ton of questions in regards to what should I put in my juicer and we thought it best if we broke it down a little and give your our results.

Skins, Stems and Seeds

When it comes to skins with juicing it's a personal preference with most produce. We've added in our recipe if you should peel an item or not.

With stems, the only stems that prove to be any beneficial for nutrients would be from grapes.

The rest of the fruits and vegetable stems you should discard as they have no nutrient value.

Removing seeds is discretionary however we recommend you do so with most produce.

Carrots

Carrots as you already know are hard little suckers so just be prepared to cut them up in half to make it easier for your juicer to extract the juices. Try not to over stuff your machine to allow the carrots enough time to be juiced. Depending on your machine you may have to use a guide/pusher to keep them from jumping all around.

Citrus Fruits

In mostly all of our recipes that contain citrus fruits we recommend you peel the skins. While they can be juiced with the skin on we ask that you remove it because the flavor can be overwhelming and can ruin the taste of the wonderful juice mix we've put together for you.

Juicing Leaves

If you haven't juiced leaves before than it is best to start off on the right foot and use this tip. When your ingredient calls for leaves, roll them in a bunch then followed by a fruit or vegetable containing a larger volume of juice such as celery, tomato, or cucumber. This will allow the leaves to be processed along with the following juicer item. (i.e baby spinach can be wrapped in a large kale leaf)

Mango, Cherries, Apricot, and Peaches

With these delicious items you want to make sure that you dispose of the pits before trying to
jam it in your juicer. You'd be surprise on how many people think it's okay to put a peach pit in their juicer.

Pineapple and mangos

These are my favorite (Jimmy) ingredients to add to any of my juices and what I've learned from them is that you need to remove the rind and cut around the mangos seed prior to juicing. If not, be prepared to do a lot of cleaning. Your juicers spout can easily get clogged by the rinds and stringy texture of these fruits if you don't remove them beforehand.

Here are some of the fruits and vegetables that are easy to juice, not so easy to juice, and the ones that give you the most juice for your beverage.

Fruits and Vegetables: Easy to Juice:

Apples	Grapefruits	Peaches
Asparagus	Grapes	Pears
Brussels sprouts	Guava	Peppers
Cabbages	Honeydew Melon	Pomegranate seeds
Cantaloupe	Horseradish	Potatoes
Celery	Kiwi	Pumpkin
Cherries (pitted)	Lemon	Radicchio
Clementines	Lettuces	Radishes
Cranberries	Lime	Squashes
Cucumber	Nectarines	Strawberries
Fennel	Onion	Tangerines
Garlic	Oranges	Tomatoes
Ginger	Parsnip	Watermelon

Fruits and Vegetables: Not as Easy to Juice

Apricot	Kale	Pears
Basil	Leafy greens	Peppermint
Beets	Leeks	Pineapple
Blackberries	Mango	Plums
Blueberries	Mint	Raspberries
Broccoli	Mushroom	Spinach
Carrots	Mustard greens	Swiss chard
Cauliflower	Nectarines	Tomatoes
Collard greens	Okra	Turnip
Dandelion greens	Papaya	Watercress

Endive	Parsley	Wheat grass
Green beans	Passion fruit	
Green peas	Peaches	

Fruits and Vegetables: Juicy Juice! These will fill your cup up quickly.

Apples	Cucumber	Lime
Cantaloupe	Grapefruits	Oranges
Celery	Grapes	Peppers
Clementines	Honeydew Melon	Pineapple
Cranberries	Lemon	Tangerines
Tomatoes	Watermelon	

3 Day Vegetarian Meal Plan (Bonus #3)

As a reward for completing your cleanse and to show our appreciation, we have created a 3 day nutritional plan to follow to ease you back into consuming whole foods. This meal plan is free of wheat, gluten, soy and preservatives.
Please drink plenty of water with this meal plan and avoid diet drinks, processed fruit drinks and sodas.

<u>**Shopping list:**</u>
1 package of steel cut oats
1 carton of rice or almond milk
Brown sugar
Sliced almonds
Herbal tea of choice
3 cups of blueberries
3 cups of organic plain yogurt
5 red beets
3 avocados (optional)
Balsamic vinegar
1 bunch or large container of arugula
1 packet of walnuts
1 packet of dried cranberries
1 container of feta cheese
3 bananas
1 container of protein powder
2 cans of black beans
Cilantro
Parsley
Red pepper flakes
Salt and Pepper
Tortilla chips (baked or fried, your choice)
Pepper jack cheese
Tomatillo or Enchilada Sauce (1 can is enough if buying pre-made)

1 small onion
1 egg
Almond meal

Breakfast: *Approx 305 calories*
Steel cut oatmeal - add rice or almond milk, 1 teaspoon of organic brown sugar and sliced almonds
Herbal tea or freshly pressed fruit juice
Follow cooking instructions on carton of oatmeal. Add remaining ingredients once finished cooking.

Mid morning snack: *Approx 230 calories if choosing whole milk yogurt*
1 cup of fresh blueberries with 1 cup of organic plain yogurt
Mix and enjoy

Lunch: *Approx 470 calories. Add 300 calories with 1 sliced avocado over the salad.*
Roasted red beet and arugula salad - (prepare the night before) - roast 5 beets in the oven, serve 1-2 red beets peeled & diced, over arugula with ¼ cup of walnuts, ¼ cup feta cheese, ¼ cup dried cranberries, balsamic vinegar. Use remaining red beets and ingredients for another salad.

Afternoon snack: *Calories vary depending on brand of protein powder used*
Protein smoothie - blend 1 banana with 1 cup of rice milk and 1 or 2 scoops of your favorite protein powder.

Dinner: *Approx 950 calories for whole casserole. Makes approx 4 servings (237 calories per serving)*
Black bean enchilada bake - Food process 2 cans of black beans (drained and rinsed), mix with 1 small finely chopped onion, 1 small bunch of cilantro chopped, 1 small bunch of parsley chopped, 1 tablespoon of red pepper flakes, 1 tablespoon of salt, 1 tablespoon of pepper, 1 minced garlic clove, 1 egg, ¼ cup of almond meal.
Layer a casserole dish with tomatillo sauce or red enchilada sauce, 1 layer of tortilla chips, black bean mixture and top with 1 layer of tortilla chips, remaining sauce, and a small sprinkle of pepper jack cheese.
Bake on 350 degrees for 40 minutes.

Conclusion

This concludes your 3 day detoxification.

Now that you're finished with this book you have the skills necessary to properly detox all the while picking out the best fruit and vegetable combo (organic and nonorganic) that will fit your taste and juicing goals.

You've also learned:

What to look for when choosing your ingredients

- The different types of juicers to choose from

- What cleaning tools and utensils that you should have in your arsenal

- How to map out the best time to start your detox regimen

- How to create a shopping list based on what you enjoy

- How to plan for the "before, during, and after" stages

- and so much more other than just recipes...

Thank you again for taking your personal time out to read our book(s) and following through with your detox. Now with that said we can happily announce that you are now Officially part of the Juice Fam team. **Congrats!!**

Our early Juice Fam friends and family that have gotten their hands on this book before we made it public has tremendously helped us out by telling us what they wanted to know more of, what they liked or disliked, and we've added as much of it in here for you as we could. So....

Your Next Steps

Write us an honest review about what you thought about this book – We truly value your opinion and thoughts. **Five star** reviews will help us spread the word and also allow us to become better writers and make updates to our previous work.

Please leave your review by clicking here:

AMAZON

⭐⭐⭐⭐⭐

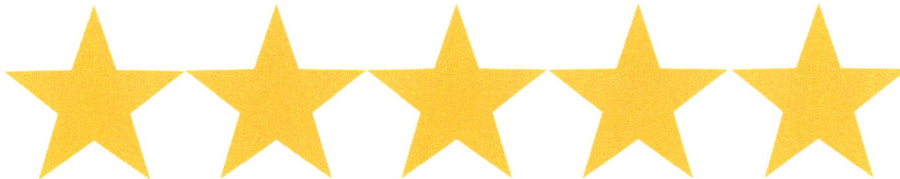

Please Give Us Your Honest Review
(http://www.juicefam.com/review)

Check out our recommendations for more juicing tips and recipes.
Here are some books that others who've bought ours have also purchased.

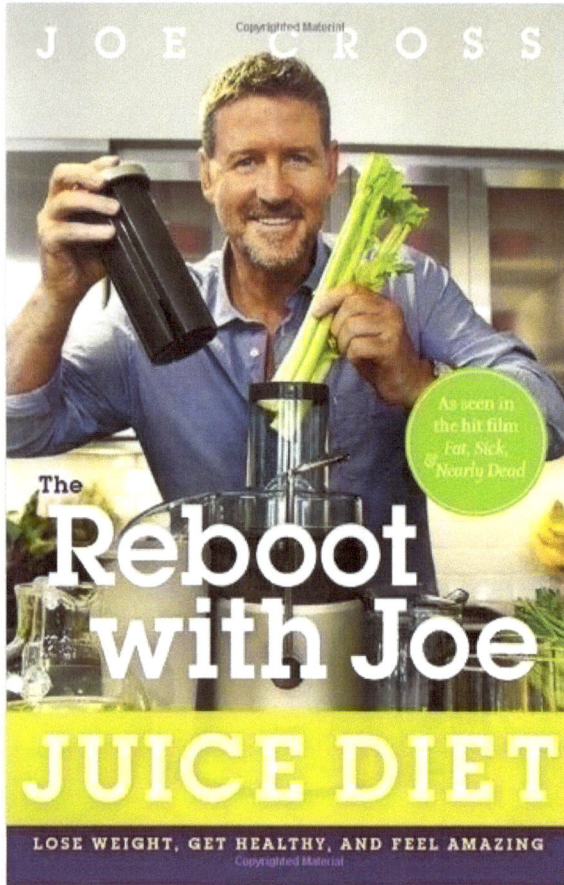

The Reboot with Joe Juice Diet: Lose Weight, Get Healthy, And Feel Amazing

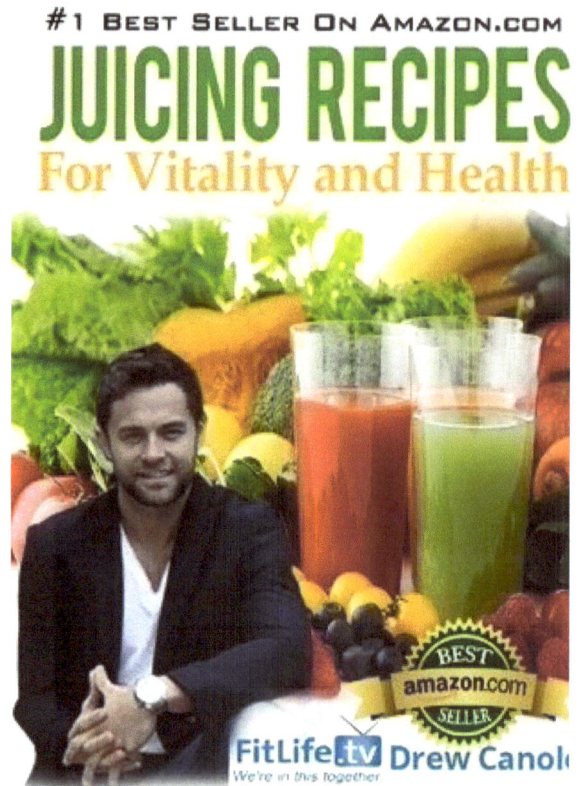

Juicing Recipes From Fitlife.TV Star Drew Canole For Vitality and Health

Last note, Melissa and James personally know what it's like to change bad habits and with you accomplishing your 3 day detox goal as they have you'll be way ahead of the game on other parts of your life that you want to change as well.

So go out there, live life, juice, and be healthy.

Cheers from the Juice Fam Team,

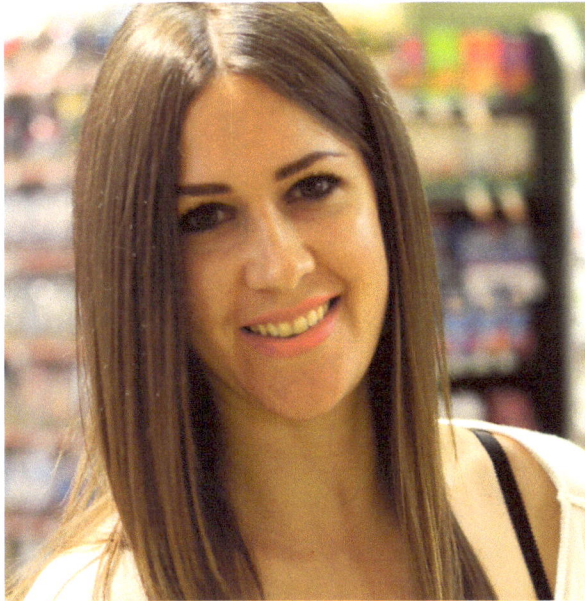

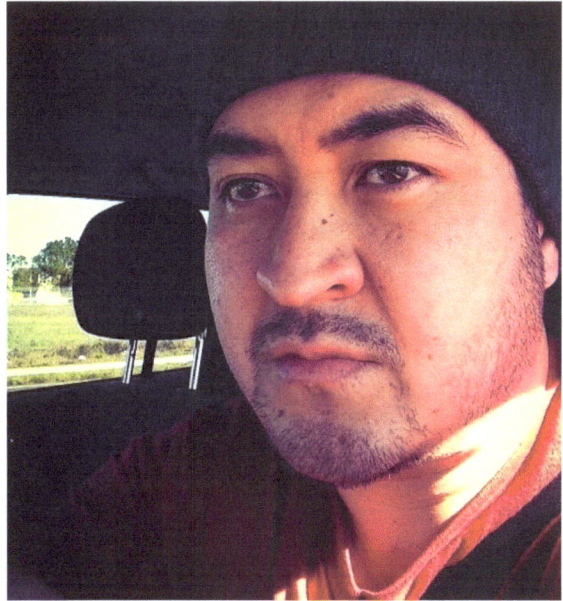

Melissa Bell and James Delong

P.S. Don't forget to get your **FREE** juicing recipes and become one of our VIP's by heading over to

http://www.juicefam.com/free-updates today!

P.P.S. Please don't forget to leave us a review.

www.JuiceFam.com/Review